Cardio-Vascular Diseases since Harvey's Discovery

THE
HARVEIAN ORATION

Cardio-Vascular Diseases since Harvey's Discovery

THE
HARVEIAN ORATION

Delivered before
The Royal College of Physicians
of London

on

18 October 1928

By

SIR HUMPHRY DAVY ROLLESTON

*Bart., K.C.B., M.A., M.D., Hon. D.Sc.,
D.C.L., LL.D.*

*Fellow and sometime President of the Royal
College of Physicians of London
Physician in Ordinary to the King
Regius Professor of Physic
Cambridge*

CAMBRIDGE

AT THE UNIVERSITY PRESS

1928

CAMBRIDGE
UNIVERSITY PRESS

University Printing House, Cambridge CB2 8BS, United Kingdom

Published in the United States of America by Cambridge University Press, New York

Cambridge University Press is part of the University of Cambridge.

It furthers the University's mission by disseminating knowledge in the pursuit of education, learning and research at the highest international levels of excellence.

www.cambridge.org
Information on this title: www.cambridge.org/9781107660854

© Cambridge University Press 1928

First published 1928
First paperback edition 2014

A catalogue record for this publication is available from the British Library

ISBN 978-1-107-66085-4 Paperback

....

To

SIR JOHN ROSE BRADFORD

K.C.M.G., C.B., C.B.E., M.D., D.SC. (*London*), F.R.S.
President of the Royal College of Physicians
of London; Emeritus Professor of
Medicine, University College,
and Consulting Physician
to University College
Hospital

CONTENTS

INTRODUCTION

THE PRESIDENT'S command to deliver the 272nd Harveian Oration in the tercentenary year of the publication of the *Exercitatio Anatomica de Motu Cordis et Sanguinis in Animalibus* is an honour to be prized with humble gratitude, but with a due sense of its heavy responsibility, by any man, especially by one whose father obeyed the call to this high duty fifty-five years ago.

Harvey, the acknowledged Father of modern physiology, returned to the Greek method of experiment which had been in almost complete abeyance since the time of Claudius Galen (A.D. 130–200), "the first Father of experimental physiology", whose authority and teaching had remained sacrosanct for more than thirteen hundred years. The tercentenary of the publication of Harvey's immortal discovery in the work described by Albrecht von Haller as "Opusculum aureum" was appropriately and splendidly commemorated by the celebrations organized by this College. In no way could its significance have been more suitably and graphically shown than by the remarkable cinematograph films of Harvey's original physiological experiments as repeated by Sir Thomas Lewis and Dr H. H. Dale, Fellows of the College, who have been eminent in obedience to Harvey's exhortation "to search and study out the secrets of nature by way of experiment". Further, the historical aspect of the tercentenary has been permanently marked by the College in the production of a facsimile of the first edition of the *De Motu Cordis*, and by the appearance of two other Harveian books, a reproduction of the first English translation in 1653 of the *De Motu Cordis* (Nonesuch Press), and *A Bibliography of the Writings of William Harvey, M.D.* (Cambridge University Press), both due to the pious devotion of a licentiate of the College, Mr Geoffrey Keynes.

John Freind (1675–1728), the elegant scholar and eminent physician, when commenting on the history of the circulation, wrote in 1725: "From this discovery of our great countryman (Harvey) many improvements, even in the cure of distempers, might be made: he had thoughts of composing such a work himself, to show the advantages of this doctrine, in relation to practice, but was prevented by sickness and death: the design of the Architect was very noble, and I with some of his successors might finish it. At present I shall hint only at two or three particulars, which will convince us, of what use a perfect knowledge of the circulation may be to us, if rightly applied, in the practical part of our profession". He then points out that bleeding vessels in an amputation or other wound should be

ligatured and not painfully cauterized, that in cases
of aneurysm the vessel should be tied in preference
to compression, and that the discussion which had
lasted almost two centuries, whether in pleurisy a
vein should be pricked on the same or on the
opposite side, was futile. If more than two centuries
ago the learned author of *The History of Physick from
the Time of Galen to the beginning of the xvi Century* apparently thought the task difficult and accordingly
acted with wise discretion, it is now obviously, from
limitations of both time and capacity, impossible to
attempt more than the barest outline of the accumu-
lated knowledge of the diseases of the circulatory
system since Harvey's time. A course which recalls
the self-administered reproach of Thomas Tenison
(1636–1715) when giving "a true and plain account"
of Francis Bacon's works: "Sometimes mean men
get a stock of reputation by gathering up the *Frag-
ments of the Learned*; as Beggars (they say) have
gotten estates by saving together *The Alms of the
Rich*". An attempt to piece together the history of
the various forms of cardiac disease is attended by
no small difficulties: it often happens that the same
ideas occur to several minds at the same time but
that simultaneous and identical solutions are not
published synchronously, thus making it far from
easy to decide who really deserves the rather barren
crown of priority. Another obvious objection to

such a subject is that it entails lists of men and dates; but as many of these names are those of Fellows of this College it will surely be in obedience to Harvey's injunction to commemorate these benefactors of the College, for can any benefaction be more welcome than new and true knowledge?

REFERENCES

FLINT, H. L. The Heart: Old and New Views. London, 1921. (A useful review of the whole history.)

FREIND, J. The History of Physick from the Time of Galen to the beginning of the xvi Century. 1725. Vol. 1, p. 237.

MOON, R. O. Growth of our Knowledge of Heart Disease. London, 1927.

TENISON, T., in A Discourse by Way of Introduction to Baconia or Certain Genuine Remains of Sr Francis Bacon, p. 4. London, 1679.

History of Cardio-vascular Diseases since Harvey's Discovery

IT is impossible to estimate how much information about the diseases of the heart and vessels was lost with those works of Harvey which were either destroyed when his lodgings in Whitehall were plundered by the Roundheads in 1642 or, though designed, were never completed, such as "The Practice of Medicine conformable to the Thesis of the Circulation of the Blood", and that mentioned at the end of his second Disquisition to John Riolan in the following words: "I shall have much to put forth in my Medical Observations and Pathology which, so far as I know, has yet been observed by no one, about the innumerable diseases concerned with disturbances of the circulation and their cure".

The knowledge of cardio-vascular disease which was very slight at the time of the discovery of the circulation has since come through several channels: (1) the accumulation of data provided by anatomical observation, normal and morbid, (2) unaided clinical observation, (3) as the result of the application of instruments of precision to the examination of patients, and (4), probably most important, the in-

formation derived from physiological and pathological experiments. Though these four headings are
attractive as a means of sketching the birth and
advance of modern knowledge, it is in practice
difficult, and indeed somewhat inconvenient, to
follow them out rigidly or attempt to make them
absolutely watertight; there will therefore be much
overlapping, as will at once be only too obvious.

I
Anatomical Observation

Anatomy is an indispensable step to the more complex science of physiology which explains the vital
forces of the body and this, though it may be helped
by anatomy, demands observation of or experiment
on the living organism. Fabricius' description of the
valves in the veins stimulated Harvey to find out
their use by the experimental method. Gaskell's
physiological demonstration of the muscular continuity between the auricle and the ventricle was
made on reptiles and was supposed to be confined
to them until 1893, when the auriculo-ventricular
bundle was described in mammals by Stanley Kent
and by W. His, junior; in 1906 Tawara gave a full
account of the junctional system, including the
auriculo-ventricular node and the bundle previously
described by Kent and His, the fibres of the bundle
being continued into the Purkinje fibres which line

the interior of the ventricles and communicate with their muscular fibres; this was followed in 1907 by Keith and Flack's discovery of the sino-auricular node, the normal pace-maker of the mammalian heart; the later anatomical observations were subsequent to and directly stimulated by the needs of the new cardiology, for Mackenzie's epoch-making book on the pulse was published in 1902. Thus it may be noted that, just as medicine is deeply indebted to the experimental method, so also science owes a debt to medicine, and that they two "according well may make one music as before".

The capillaries. It must have been an almost insuperable obstacle to the conception of the circulation that the arteries and veins gradually diminishing in size ended in the tissues without any visible communications. The probability of some continuity had been rather vaguely foreshadowed by Aristotle and Erasistratus, and it was assumed that there were direct communications between the arteries and veins, resembling in miniature what is now known as an arterio-venous aneurysm, and indeed the direct communication between the coronary arteries and the Thebesian vessels recently shown by Wearn. This was the view held in the seventeenth century by Riolan, Cornelius ab Hogeland, and Descartes.

Henry Power (1623–68), the author of *Experimental Philosophy, in three Books, containing new Ex-*

periments, Microscopical, Mercurial and Magnetical, 1664, was a correspondent of Sir Thomas Browne and, as his subsequent letters show, took heed of the advice, probably given him in 1647 when at Cambridge, to make himself "master of Dr Harvey's piece *De Circul. Sang.*" In an unpublished manuscript (1663, Sloane MS. 1343) in the British Museum, for a transcript of which I am much indebted to Dr Charles Singer, Power describes how, although using Leeuwenhoek's lens, he could never detect any opening between the arteries and veins, though in a letter to Sir Thomas Browne in 1649 he speaks of "the minute and capillary chanells". Richard Lower in his *Tractatus de Corde,* 1669, inferred that there were hair-like tubes too small to be seen uniting the arteries and veins. The tercentenary of the birth of Marcello Malpighi, the father of histology, on 10 March 1628 and that of the *De Motu* appropriately coincide, for in 1661 he provided the final proof of Harvey's discovery by recognizing the capillaries in the frog's lung. He also saw the red blood corpuscles in the mesenteric vessels of a hedgehog, but as he regarded them as fat cells, Antony van Leeuwenhoek, "the immortal Bedell" as B. Ward Richardson christened him, who described them fully in his *True Circulation of the Blood* in 1686, has the credit of their recognition. Johannes Swammerdam, however, had actually noted the presence of red blood cells as early as 1658, but his observation was not made public until 1738 when Boerhaave brought out Swammerdam's *Biblia Naturae*. Luciani gives the credit of first seeing with a microscope the red corpuscles in the capillaries of a living animal (an embryo chick) to Lazzaro Spallanzani in 1771.

After the discovery of the capillaries there was a long interval before this most essential part of the circulatory system received due attention. Thomas Young in 1808 had the foresight to assume as probable variation in the size of the capillaries. Poiseuille in 1834 noticed the central core of red cells and the peripheral layer of plasma with the more slowly moving leucocytes. The view that the capillary circulation was a mere passive communication between the arterioles and the venules was definitely modified by Stricker's observation in 1865 that the capillaries became constricted from swelling of the endothelial cells. In 1873 Rouget observed on the surface of capillaries the cells which bear his name, and described their contraction; this was confirmed by Vimtrup and by Krogh; but Aschoff and Ohno disputed this and regarded them as adventitial cells, a view endorsed by Clark and Clark, who observed contraction of the capillary endothelium both before the Rouget cells appear and in areas devoid of Rouget cells when these have developed. In 1879 Roy and

Graham Brown showed that the calibre of the
capillaries is constantly changing without corresponding alterations in the arteriolar pressure. The
study of the capillary circulation then languished;
but the invention of capillary microscopy by
Lombard in 1912 again stimulated investigation, and
it has now been proved that the walls of the capillaries have independent powers of changing their
calibre. The mechanism of variations in the size of
the capillaries—their dilatation and constriction—
has been much discussed; there are obviously several
possibilities: what share is played respectively by
the direct action on the capillaries of the vasomotor
nerves discovered by Claude Bernard in 1851, by
chemical influence, and mechanically by the conditions of the circulation in the arterioles and
venules? In a review of the subject in 1921 Hooker
concludes that while the capillary bed responds to
both chemical and nervous influences, the chemical
are concerned with dilatation and the nervous with
constriction.

The capillary circulation, thanks to the experimental labours of Dale, Laidlaw, Richards, Krogh,
and Lewis, has been placed in a new light. It appears
that the capillary area as a whole is in a constant
state of flux; while the great portion is relatively
empty, various parts of it open for a time, so that
with a constantly changing condition of the con-

stituent portions the average total path remains
about the same and maintains the peripheral resistance. Normally only a very small proportion of
the whole available capillary area is open, for if it
were universally open all the blood would stagnate
there. The varying dilatation of the capillaries
corresponds, as Krogh demonstrated in muscle,
with the needs for it. Dale and his co-workers showed that histamine exerts a toxic action on capillary
endothelium, producing dilatation of the lumen and
increased permeability of the walls of the capillary
while constricting the arterioles. Inchley (1926),
however, describes the capillary dilatation as a
passive mechanical result of constriction of the
veins, which are more sensitive than the arteries to
the action of histamine. Lewis and his collaborators
have shown that slight local damage to the skin
causes dilatation of the capillaries, which they argued
may be due to the liberation of a histamine-like body.
In 1919 Dale suggested that while the course of
adjustment of the blood supply to organs or considerable areas of the body may well be under
nervous control, the fine adjustment of the capillary
circulation within these areas may be due to small
quantities of a histamine-like body.

From observations on animals with histamine
poisoning light has been thrown on the causation
of shock, whether traumatic or bacterial. In ex-

tensive damage of the soft tissues a histamine-like body would, it appears probable, be produced and lead to widespread dilatation of the capillaries so that the blood stagnates there at the expense of the rest of the vascular system, and further that the blood plasma passes into the tissues and thus oligaemia results. Similarly in acute infections a poison may be formed which acts like histamine, so that blood collects in the capillaries and is concentrated by the escape of the plasma into the tissues.

The question whether the circulation in the nervous system, the lungs, and the coronary vessels is under the same nervous control as the rest of the general systemic capillaries has been exhaustively investigated and is referred to briefly elsewhere; the effect of adrenaline on the vessels—constriction or its absence—has been employed as a criterion of the presence or absence of vasomotor fibres, but can hardly, for example, in the case of the coronary arteries (*vide* p. 126), be regarded as devoid of exceptions due to a species difference in the nerve supply and reactions (*vide* Anrep).

Morbid anatomy must also be supplemented by clinical observation or by experiment; the example set by Harvey of always submitting to the test of physiological proof the explanations suggested by anatomy, which is completely instructive only when elucidated by physiological experiment, was followed with regard to morbid anatomy and its correlation with symptoms by Morgagni, Corvisart, Laennec, Hope, and later the experimental results obtained by Claude Bernard, Cohnheim, Roy, Starling, and many others were brought to supplement the teaching of the post-mortem room.

It was not until the eighteenth century, with the publication of observations on morbid anatomy made by Raymond Vieussens (1715), Lancisi (1718, 1740), and Morgagni (1761), and the first treatise dealing specially with diseases of the heart by J. B. de Senac (1749), that cardiac disease was really recognized. Theophilus Bonetus[1] (1620–89), in the first volume of his *Sepulchretum* (1679), collected a number of observations on palpitation and cardiac pain during life associated with polypi in the heart, calculi in the myocardium, inflammation of the heart, acute inflammation, effusion and adhesion of the pericardium, and aortic aneurysm, and thus prepared the way for Morgagni and others. Vieussens and Morgagni recorded a number of valvular lesions, and Lancisi[2] in 1718 described vegetations

[1] Bonetus, T., *Sepulchretum sive Anatomica practica ex Cadaveribus morbo denatis, proponens Historias et Observationes omnium humani Corporis affectuum, ipsorumque Causas reconditas revelans*, 1679, I, 816.

[2] Lancisi, J. M., *De subitaneis Mortibus*, 1718. *De Motu Cordis et Aneurysmatibus*, 1740.

on the valves and noted dilatation and hypertrophy, but applied the term aneurysm to the former; in his posthumous book (1740) syphilitic lesions of the heart were outlined. De Senac[1] described ulceration, abscess, and inflammation of the heart, "the hairy heart" of acute pericarditis, and in a short chapter malformations.

Corvisart and his pupils, Laennec and Bouillaud, carried on the anatomico-clinical investigation of cardiac affections, and among the Fellows of this College James Hope (1801–41) set a fine example in this respect.

ANATOMICO-CLINICAL HISTORY OF VARIOUS CARDIO-VASCULAR DISEASES

There is naturally a considerable difference both chronologically and in practical importance between the earliest descriptions of morbid lesions of the heart and their clinical recognition. But in order to minimize repetition some details of the clinical recognition will be combined with the earliest anatomical records of the various cardiac lesions.

DISEASES OF THE PERICARDIUM

Raymond Vieussens in 1706 recorded the morbid appearances of pericardial adhesions and diagnostic

[1] De Senac, J. B., *Traité de la structure du cœur, de son action et ses maladies*, 1749, ed. 2, 1783, vol. II, p. 305.

signs of effusion into the pericardium. Joseph
Exupère Bertin is quoted in 1824 by his son as
having observed a case of acute pericarditis in 1739,
but the first published account of the disease was by
de Senac in 1749. Laennec described some of the
physical signs of acute pericarditis, but stated that
"of all the severe lesions of the thoracic organs
three alone remain without pathognomonic signs to
a practitioner expert in auscultation and percussion
—namely, aortic aneurysm, pericarditis, and polypi
in the heart previous to death". Collin in 1824 was
the first to give an adequate account of pericardial
friction, which he compared to the creaking of new
leather. Andral in 1829 recorded pericarditis in
acute rheumatism, and in 1839 Bright said that he
had long been aware of the association of pericarditis with chorea.

The early history of the operative treatment of
the pericardial effusion is fully given by Trousseau
and Lasègue. John Riolan the younger suggested
that it should be done, as did Senac and others.
Desault in 1798 unsuccessfully attempted it, and
writing in 1819 Mérat quoted three cases, two
followed by recovery, which were punctured by
Romero of Barcelona. In 1840 Schuh of Vienna
operated, as in 1841 did Heger, also of Vienna, on
a case with effusions into the pericardium, both
pleurae and peritoneum associated with tuberculosis.

A case of Trousseau's was operated upon in 1854, and in this country paracentesis of the pericardium was done on two cases under the care of Clifford Allbutt (1868). Samuel West in 1883 recorded a case in which he twice tapped and then successfully drained a purulent pericarditis, and collected eighty cases of paracentesis or drainage of the pericardium.

Universally adherent pericardium with much fibrosis, which may involve the chest wall and in extreme instances the adjacent tissues so as to constitute chronic indurative mediastino-pericarditis, as Kussmaul named it in 1873, is often combined with valvular disease; but even without this added factor it may be responsible for cardiac insufficiency and failure. Morgagni, Senac, other early observers, and Corvisart considered adherent pericardium a serious handicap; Laennec and Hope failed to confirm Sander's signs of alteration in the state of the chest wall in the praecordial region. Hope in 1839 described as new signs the normal position of the enlarged heart as if braced up by adhesions, a prominence of the praecordial costal cartilages, and a jogging or tumbling motion of the heart during systole and diastole, as if its action were suddenly arrested. C. J. B. Williams (1840) could not confirm the "jogging" motion, but pointed out the widespread pulsation of the chest wall, and the unchanging cardiac dullness on inspiration and expiration; Sibson (1844) and Bouillaud (1846) re-cognized retraction of the praecordial region, and Skoda in 1852 further emphasized the systolic recession. Griesinger, as reported by Widenmann in 1856, observed in a case of chronic mediastino-pericarditic fibrosis the pulse intermitting during respiration, which in 1873 Kussmaul called the para-doxical pulse, and ascribed to compression of the aortic arch by adhesions at each inspiration. Wilks in 1871 directed special attention to the cardiac aspect of adherent pericardium. Adherent peri-cardium may be combined with a chronic inflam-matory condition of the two pleurae and of the peritoneum, polyserositis, polyorrhymenitis, or Concato's disease (Heidemann, Gilbert and Garnier, F. Taylor) which imitates chronic peritonitis. Adherent pericardium may be associated with a high degree of chronic venous engorgement of the liver and recurrent ascites but with little or no chronic peritonitis or hepatitis; this was described by Pick in 1896 as pericarditic pseudo-cirrhosis of the liver. Calcification of an adherent pericardium was re-corded by Bonetus and Morgagni, and since 1910 has been recognized by X-rays (Schwarz). Retrac-tion of the tenth and eleventh interspaces below the left scapula and due to adhesions between the heart, pericardium and diaphragm, was described in 1895 by John Broadbent, and is known as Broadbent's sign.

Primary *new growths* of the pericardium are almost unknown, cases so described, such as that of W. Broadbent, must be distinguished from those primary in the adjacent thymus. Metastases of either sarcoma or carcinoma elsewhere are not very uncommon, and direct extension from intrathoracic growths, but not from the oesophagus, occur (Douglas).

DISEASES OF THE MYOCARDIUM

The striking changes of hypertrophy and dilatation did not escape the notice of the early pathologists, Nicolas Massa being said to have noted hypertrophy in 1534. But, though they attracted the attention of Laennec and of Bertin and Bouillaud (1824), knowledge of the nature of myocardial lesions had necessarily to await the era of histological examination. In spite of the stress laid by Corvisart (1806) on the importance of the myocardium and of the dictum of his pupil Laennec that it was "the key to cardiac pathology", which his followers Hope and Clendinning later echoed, the adoption of auscultation focussed attention on valvular murmurs which were first regarded as evidence of irreparable damage—a verdict subsequently partially lightened by the admission of functional or inorganic murmurs. This lasted during the greater part of the last century and was responsible for neglect of myocardial diseases, which in 1809, before the advent of auscultation, had been declared by Allan Burns to be less frequent than those of the valves. It should, however, be remembered that W. Stokes in 1854 insisted that the symptoms associated with evidence of valvular disease depended on the state of the myocardium and not on the valvular lesions.

Laennec described as softening what would now be called toxic myocarditis in the infective fevers. Bouillaud, Louis, and Andral who in 1826 regarded the knowledge of heart disease as almost complete, also scrutinized the naked-eye appearances of the heart in fevers, but mainly noted changes in colour and consistency of the muscle; and Stokes in 1834 studied the softening of the myocardium in typhus, correlating it with physical signs.

Hope's views on the causation of dilatation and hypertrophy of the heart are practically those now current, namely, that dilatation follows regurgitation into the cardiac cavity, and is also due to softening and insufficiency of the myocardium, and that hypertrophy is the result of increased work, such as obstruction to the exit of blood from the cavity. Hope first made clear the influence of regurgitation, for until then the hypertrophy and dilatation were explained as opposite responses to obstruction to the exit of blood from the affected cavities. It may be added that Hope in 1839 had seen many examples of cardiac hypertrophy in Oxford and Cambridge oarsmen.

Fatty degeneration. Corvisart was much interested in fatty infiltration, and Laennec described fatty degeneration of the heart. The fatty degeneration in pernicious anaemia was described by Coombe and Kellie in 1824, but escaped general attention, and was pointed out again forty years later by Dickinson. Peacock, James Paget (1847), Ormerod (1849), and Richard Quain (1850) were largely responsible for the recognition of fatty degeneration of the myocardium in this country; Paget both by his own observations and by making known Rokitansky's work (1844), and Quain, who credited Lancisi with having seen it, by careful pathological research. Stokes specially correlated with fatty degeneration of the heart the well-known type of breathing first described by John Cheyne in 1816, and known under their combined names, and the syndrome afterwards called that of Stokes-Adams. In the thyrotoxic heart of Graves' disease and adenomatous goitre with hyperthyroidism, in which auricular flutter and fibrillation may occur, fatty degeneration of the myocardium is common (Wilson).

Fibroid disease. Corvisart in 1806 described gross changes—induration—which may have been fibroid disease, but as late as 1838 little was known about this condition now so important in connection with its effects on the junctional system; Hope in his treatise devotes but three-quarters of a page to "induration of the heart" and quotes Bertin and Bouillaud's opinion that it is one of the products of chronic inflammation. Richard Quain exhibited a specimen before the Pathological Society of London in 1850, and Wilks in 1857 suggested a syphilitic origin. Fagge in 1874 recorded eleven cases and collected nineteen from the *Transactions of the Pathological Society of London*. Weigert in 1880 described infarction of the heart wall as the antecedent of fibroid disease, and in 1882 Huber made it clear that coronary disease was the responsible factor. Although in 1854 Gairdner recorded a case of "ossification of the coronary arteries with tendinous degeneration of the heart", the importance of the association was not realized in this country until F. C. Turner's paper in 1881; this sequence of events was later emphasized by Steven (1887).

Cardiac aneurysm. Though originally employed in the sense now universally understood, the word aneurysm was used for general enlargement of the cardiac cavities by Lancisi, Albertini, Corvisart, Andral, and Bouillaud; Corvisart speaking of hypertrophy with dilatation as active aneurysm, and simple dilatation as passive aneurysm of the heart. Real cardiac aneurysm, then designated as partial

aneurysm of the heart, was first mentioned by
Galeati in 1751, soon afterwards by John Hunter,
and later by Matthew Baillie, who, however, in
1818 had seen it once only. Breschet in 1827 collected ten cases; in 1838 Thurnam brought together
seventy-four examples with some additional ones of
aneurysm of the valves, and Wickham Legg in 1883
collected ninety more cases since 1840 in his scholarly
Bradshaw Lecture. Rokitansky explained the
frequency of aneurysm at the apex of the heart by
the liability of this area to be attacked by chronic
myocarditis, and so correlated fibroid disease with
aneurysm.

Acute cardiac aneurysms may be secondary to
malignant endocarditis, and as a result of suppura-
tion what are apparently dissecting aneurysms of the
heart may result. Hektoen describes cases due to
acute infection of the aortic valves. In 1897 Vestberg collected sixty cases of dissecting cardiac
aneurysms; aneurysms of the sinuses of Valsalva and
the commencement of the aorta may extend into the
heart and dissect the interventricular or interauricular
septa or the walls of the ventricles.

Mechanical strain. The association of cardiac hypertrophy with renal disease was noted in 1827 by
R. Bright, who in 1836 ascribed it to the altered
character of the blood either (i) exciting the heart to
more vigorous contractions, or (ii) causing ob-

struction in the capillaries. Bertin and Laennec noticed and Hope agreed that there was a special association between hypertrophy of the left ventricle and cerebral haemorrhage, without, however, any mention of the condition of the kidneys. Much later, and just before Gull and Sutton's arterio-capillary fibrosis became public, it was suggested by Traube (1872) that excessive eating was responsible for left ventricular hypertrophy, thus anticipating hyperpiesia and essential hypertension.

The effect of excessive physical exertion on the cardio-vascular system was raised in 1839 by Hope in reference to athletics and climbing; thus he stated that boat-racing at Oxford and Cambridge, violent gymnastics and hare-and-hounds at schools have caused "rupture and inflammation of the valves and aorta, issuing in incurable organic disease....I have also repeatedly known pedestrian tours amongst the Swiss and Scotch mountains to be followed by hypertrophy and other diseases of the heart. It is protracted efforts that are always the most pernicious. Feats of this kind should always be discouraged". This of course sounds a very exaggerated statement now, but it probably left its mark on the lay, if not on the professional, mind. In 1864 Peacock drew attention to the cardiac failure in Cornish miners who not only had their hard work in the mines but were obliged to climb long distances at the end of the

day. In 1870 Clifford Allbutt wrote the first of his
three articles on the subject—"The effects of over-
work and strain on the heart and great blood vessels".
He gave examples of mitral and aortic incompetence
and of aneurysm thus caused; dilatation of the right
heart he regarded as an early result of long-continued exertion, whereas sudden strain tells more
especially on the aortic area. Roy and Adami's experimental results (1888) lent support to Allbutt's
thesis; they also showed that acute narrowing of the
aorta produced oedematous changes in those parts
of the aortic, mitral, and tricuspid valves which are
found to be thickened in abnormally high blood
pressure, and it was therefore argued that chronic
thickening of the cardiac valves may be due to
mechanical strain. Adami (1911) emphasized this
view by comparing it with the nodose endarteritis
often seen in the elderly in association with chronic
thickening of the valves, the two processes being
identical. William Collier of Oxford, an athlete of
distinction, threw out a warning of the evil effects,
though delayed for years, of excessive athleticism.
J. E. Morgan, however, in his analysis of the first
twenty-four Oxford and Cambridge boat races from
1829 to 1869, both inclusive, in which he obtained
information from all the 255 living members of the
crews except four, showed that there is little appre-
ciable difference in the mortality from heart disease

among university oarsmen and other men of a corresponding age. In his two subsequent articles (1898, 1909) Allbutt admitted that the influence of toxic and infective factors, such as alcohol, rheumatism, and syphilis, may sometimes be difficult to disentangle, and in both of them he concluded with the wise caution that "the importance of muscular effort as a factor in cardiac injury has been much exaggerated".

The condition described at various times as the *irritable heart in soldiers* (Myers (1870), Da Costa (1871)), *disordered action of the heart* (D.A.H.), and recently as *effort syndrome* (Lewis), was regarded sixty years ago as due to over-exertion; but it is now clear that the etiological factors vary and that among these cases some are infective or toxic in origin and so may be analogous to the thyrotoxic heart of exophthalmic goitre, though the condition was not one of hyperthyroidism. Collective investigation of these cases during the war showed that the condition was not primarily cardiac and that it was largely a neurosis and was adversely affected by digitalis. Though specially prominent during war time it is also seen in times of peace.

Rheumatic myocarditis was very slow to attract attention; in 1886 Hilton Fagge, like Hope in 1839, mentioned acute rheumatism as an occasional cause of cardiac hypertrophy, and in Wilks' *Lectures on*

Pathological Anatomy, in which many subsequent discoveries may be found, a belief in acute general myocarditis of rheumatic origin is expressed. In his Lumleian lectures on heart inflammation in children in 1894 Sturges resuscitated the term carditis, applied by Corvisart and Bouillaud (1841) to the combination of pericarditis and endocarditis, but he did not mean pancarditis or realize that the myocardium is affected except as a secondary result of pericarditis and especially an adherent pericardium. Sansom, Graham Steell, D. B. Lees and Poynton were among the first to believe on clinical grounds that the rheumatic poison caused myocardial inadequacy.

The submiliary nodules in the myocardium, now generally regarded as pathognomonic of acute rheumatism are the same as the subcutaneous nodules described by Hillier in 1863 and more fully in 1881 by Barlow and Warner, who pointed out their association with grave and progressive cardiac lesions. In the myocardium they were first observed as "multiple foci of small-celled exudation scattered through the walls of the ventricle", and figured by Poynton who was concerned to show that rheumatic myocarditis was not necessarily an extension from pericarditis. Aschoff in 1904 gave a fuller description of them, and they are commonly known as Aschoff's bodies. Carey Coombs also described them in detail and, like Aschoff and Tawara, failed to find them in other infections.

The alcoholic heart or dilatation due to beer-drinking and characterized by widespread oedema, dyspnoea, enlarged liver, a mitral regurgitant murmur, and recovery on abstinence and digitalis was described in 1893 by Graham Steell, whose attention had been first called to this by William Roberts in 1879. The condition was also recognized in Leeds in the 'seventies (Allbutt). In 1893 Bauer and Bollinger found that in Munich cardiac hypertrophy was common among those who drank beer to excess.

Tumours of the myocardium are rare. The earliest recorded example of a congenital rhabdomyoma, of which in 1907 Wolbach accepted twelve only, was Billard's in 1828. Half of Wolbach's twelve cases also showed diffuse cerebral scleroses. Virchow suggested that the cases of idiopathic hypertrophy of the heart in young children, of which in 1919 Howland collected twenty cases, might be diffuse rhabdomyomas, but this view has not received any support. Many cases of primary growths have been reported, according to Beck and Thatcher 150, but there is much doubt about the authenticity of them all, for the pedunculated tumours, polypi, fibromas, and fibromyxomas of the earlier pathologists may well have been organized thrombi. Perlstein (1918), who collected thirty-one examples of primary sarcoma, was unable to find a record of the condition having been diagnosed clinically. Hope in 1839 referred to twelve cases of malignant disease, including those described by Laennec, Andral and Bayle, and Bouillaud, and stated that there were usually growths in other parts of the body. Walshe (1862) definitely pointed out the rarity of primary and the comparative frequency of secondary growths and extension from intrathoracic growths. Metastatic growths are not uncommon, and melanomas appear to be specially prone to affect the myocardium.

Hydatid cysts of the heart were reported by Morgagni (1761), by Dupuytren, Thomas Trotter (1795), Andral, and others, but some doubt exists about the nature—cysticerci or echinococci—of the earlier cases. Trotter's patient was blue, oedematous, had pulmonary apoplexy, a pleural effusion, ante-mortem clot in the right auricle, and two vesicles like hydatids near the opening of the pulmonary artery, each about the size of a large oval bean. In 1846 Griesinger collected fifteen cases, and Davaine in 1860, critically eliminating some, accepted twenty-five cases. Peacock reviewed the subject in 1877, and in 1928 Dévé analysed the literature and accepted 137 cases, of which thirty-two from Great Britain was the largest number from any one country. He agrees with Peacock, contrary to current opinion, that when affected the heart is the only site of hydatid disease in the body, and considers that the infection arrives by the coronary arteries only. Sudden death may be due to rupture and consequent embolism with the liberated cysts, or occur when the cyst is intact.

ENDOCARDITIS

Acute endocarditis with vegetations on the valves was recognized by Kreysig, Corvisart (1806), named by Bouillaud, and recorded by Andral (1829). Kreysig, in what Forbes calls "his elaborately mis-arranged book", Bertin and Bouillaud regarded them as inflammatory in origin; Corvisart, struck by their resemblance to venereal warts, ascribed a luetic origin; Laennec dissented from both these views.

The importance of *acute rheumatism* in causing cardiac disease, which is now such an urgent problem, was just becoming realized a hundred years ago. Changes in the pericardium and cardiac valves in the subjects of acute joint disease had been mentioned by Bonetus and Morgagni, but without any comment. It is usually stated that David Pitcairn (1749–1809) had taught the rheumatic origin in 1788 at St Bartholomew's Hospital, where he was physician (1780–93), and the *Dictionary of National Biography* quotes John Latham, in his treatise on gout and rheumatism, as the authority; but this cannot be

verified in the only contribution on these diseases
that John Latham appears to have made, namely,
*A Letter on Rheumatism and Gout addressed to Sir
George Baker, Bart.*, pp. 80, 1796; further, his son,
Peter Mere Latham, in his remarks on the subject
does not mention Pitcairn in this connection.
Matthew Baillie, however, in the second edition of
his classical work (1797), dedicated to David Pitcairn, refers to the latter's observations and in the
edition of 1818 definitely states that Pitcairn "is to
be considered the first person who made the observation that rheumatism attacks the heart". The
obituary notice in *The Gentleman's Magazine* (1809,
LXXIX, Part 1, 295) also gave the credit to Pitcairn,
stating that the only record of this is in Baillie's
work, and Wells, writing on "Rheumatism of the
Heart" and describing fourteen cases, definitely says
that D. Pitcairn taught this in 1788. It might be
thought somewhat remarkable that such an observation should have been made before the days of
auscultation; but it appears from the Records of the
Gloucestershire Medical Society, which, as it met in
the Fleece Inn, Rodborough, Gloucestershire, was
also spoken of as the Fleece Medical Society, that
on 29 July 1789 Edward Jenner "favoured the
Society with remarks on a disease of the heart
following acute rheumatism, illustrated by dissections". In 1805 Jenner wrote to C. H. Parry of

Bath asking for the manuscript of this paper, but as he never published anything it may have been lost and his claim for priority lacks substantiation (*vide* Jacobs). It is possible that Jenner may have communicated this to David Pitcairn; but Baillie, who probably knew Jenner as a friend of his uncle John Hunter, is silent on any share Jenner may have had. In 1809 David Dundas, Serjeant Surgeon to the King, wrote on a peculiar disease of the heart "caused by a translation of rheumatism to the chest", and in 1828 Francis Hawkins gave the Goulstonian Lectures on "Rheumatism and Some Diseases of the Heart and other Organs". In 1845 Peter Mere Latham (1789–1875) wrote "In the year 1826 I was the first to teach the students of this hospital (St Bartholomew's) the fact that whenever the heart was affected in acute rheumatism a sound different from the sound of health always accompanied its contraction. This was then a new fact". Reference to his Lumleian Lectures before the College in 1827 shows that he definitely connected pericarditis, but without mentioning endocarditis, with acute rheumatism, and stated that a "bruit de soufflet" is characteristic of pericarditis. Hope in 1831 was familiar with the frequency of rheumatic endocarditis. In 1845 Latham gave the credit for the observation that endocarditis was present after death to Jean Baptiste Bouillaud (1793–1881), who in 1836 published his "law of coincidence" between rheumatism and cardiac disease, and in 1840 stated that more than half of 300 patients with cardiac disease dated their symptoms from an attack of acute rheumatism.

Treatment. With Poynton and Paine's (1900) description of a specific streptococcus and the conception of oral sepsis originated by W. Hunter (1900) and expanded into focal sepsis by F. Billings (1906) and others, acute rheumatism has in this century come to be regarded as a result of oral, dental, tonsillar, or other local infections, and active preventive measures, such as tonsillectomy, against rheumatic heart disease are in being. Vigorous treatment with salicylates combined with sufficient alkalis to obviate acidaemia will cut short rheumatic fever and so prevent cardiac complications; but once these have begun the influence of salicylates is disappointing.

The history of the salicylate treatment of rheumatic disease is not without interest; salicin was used as a substitute for quinine in France (Blaincourt), and a little later in England (Elliotson), a hundred years ago, but had dropped out of the pharmacopoeia before 1876 when T. J. Maclagan, then of Dundee, first brought it before the medical profession as a remedy for acute rheumatism. It is true that salicylic acid had previously been employed for rheumatic fever by Buss in Basle, Stricker in Berlin, and William Broadbent at St Mary's Hospital. Maclagan, who began to use salicin in 1874, reached this therapeutic triumph by a teleological process now rather unusual; believing that acute rheumatism was, like malaria, "miasmatic" in origin, he argued that "a remedy for it would be most hopefully looked for among those plants and trees whose favourite habitat presented conditions analogous to those under which the rheumatic miasm seemed most to prevail". He therefore turned to the willow, the bark of which was known to yield salicin, and later found that the Hottentots had long employed a decoction of the shoots of the willow as a traditional remedy for rheumatic fever. The actual use of sodium salicylate was introduced by Germain Sée (1817–96) in 1877. The success of treatment by salicin and salicylic acid was shown by Hilton Fagge's analysis of 355 patients thus treated in Guy's Hospital, 1876–80. Before this time the treatment of acute rheumatism had been of various kinds, and its value, at least in the time of the otherwise cheerful Richard Warren (1731–97), may be judged by his epigrammatic answer of "six weeks" when asked what was good for acute rheumatism. Gull and Sutton, however, as the outcome of observations on twenty-five cases treated on purely expectant lines (such as peppermint water) gave a shorter period as the natural course of the disease, namely, on an average nineteen days, and showed that cardiac complications occurred within the first few days. Owen Rees (1849) believed in lemon juice, and H. W. Fuller advocated massive alkaline treatment, and insisted that besides shortening the duration of the illness it prevented cardiac disease, if the urine was made alkaline first. By the combination of alkaline treatment with salicylates D. B. Lees (1904) was able to give doses of salicylates which would otherwise have been toxic, even as much as 600 grains of salicylate and 1200 grains of bicarbonate of sodium daily.

Prolonged rest for the heart when damaged by rheumatism was first emphasized by Francis Sibson (1814–76) in 1877 and was further insisted upon by Richard Caton (1842–1926) in his Harveian Oration of 1904, after twenty years' experience.

Malignant or ulcerative endocarditis was really first described by William Senhouse Kirkes (1823–64) in 1852 in his paper on "Some of the principal effects resulting from the detachment of fibrinous deposits from the interior of the heart and their admixture with the circulating blood", his observations being independent of, though contemporaneous with, those of Virchow on embolism. He compared the condition to the secondary deposits occurring in

phlebitis after wounds. It is not difficult to detect
the presence of malignant endocarditis in cases
previously reported, for example by Corvisart (1806),
in an illustration of the aortic valves in Joseph
Hodgson's monograph (1815). Bouillaud also drew
attention to a form of acute endocarditis with
pyaemic symptoms, and a case given by Barlow and
Rees (1843) is now recognizable as subacute bacterial
endocarditis. In his Goulstonian lectures for 1851
Edward Latham Ormerod, names revered in this
College, who as his predecessor in the post-mortem
room at St Bartholomew's Hospital was in touch
with Kirkes and acknowledged information about
endocarditis from him, recorded a case of cardiac
disease with febrile paroxysms at 4 a.m. and 4 p.m.
under the observation of Professor H. J. H. Bond
at Cambridge, the necropsy showing vegetations,
some conical, others pendulous, on the valves. Elsewhere he refers to ruptured valves and chordae
tendineae, and appears to have grasped the idea of
embolism.

In 1861 Charcot and Vulpian insisted on the
typhoidal form, and in 1870 Wilks emphasized
embolism of the small vessels and, by terming the
disease arterial pyaemia, carried on Kirkes' com-
parison with venous pyaemia. Osler's Goulstonian
Lectures in 1885, based on an analysis of more than
200 cases, gave a graphic picture of the disease, which

at the time was considered to be the most complete summary of current knowledge; like Rokitansky (1855), Heilberg, Klebs, Birch-Hirschfeld and others, he observed bacteria in the vegetations, in fact finding them constantly. The liability of grossly congenitally deformed valves to become infected was first pointed out in 1844 by James Paget in recording what is now recognizable as acute gono-coccal endocarditis of the pulmonary valves; Orme-rod in 1851 quoted Paget's statement as a general law, but otherwise it appears to have been for-gotten, for in 1886 Osler independently brought out the frequency with which malignant endocarditis supervened on bicuspid aortic valves, and A. E. Garrod (1897) did the same. Recently Lewis and Grant have gone exhaustively into the presence and influence of minute abnormalities of the aortic valves, and Maude Abbott into the statistical aspect, thus proving the correctness of Paget's conception of eighty-four years ago. Thayer's fine monograph (1926) on bacterial endocarditis contains a wealth of clinical observation ranging over many years, as his description of gonococcic endocarditis in 1895 shows.

The chronic and subacute form or endocarditis maligna lenta, though mentioned by Osler in 1885, was first definitely described from a clinical aspect in 1909 by him and by Horder. By this time much work on the bacteriological side had been done; the micro-organism usually responsible was shown by Schottmüller and by Libman who described it as the *Streptococcus viridans seu mitis* and *Streptococcus endocarditidis* respectively, to be different from those found in the acute cases. The bacteria-free phase and the healing of the endocardial lesions, though death may occur from the resulting and characteristic diffuse glomerular nephritis (Baehr), were pointed out by Libman in 1913. The relation of chronic bacterial endocarditis to rheumatic endocarditis and the transitional form of malignant rheumatism (Lenhartz; Poynton and Paine) have been much discussed and recently Thayer (1926) has reviewed the subject; but there is much to be said for the view that such an apparent transition is due to superadded infection, for while Aschoff's bodies in the myocardium and subcutaneous nodules are confined to rheumatic infection, chronic bacterial endocarditis is characterized by their absence and the presence of a round-celled interstitial lesion (Bracht-Waechter) in the myocardium, Osler's nodes, and diffuse glomerular nephritis.

The European War brought out the relative frequency of subacute and chronic bacterial endocarditis among soldiers, without any known antecedent cardiac disease, who had been exposed to much physical strain and various infections. The recognition of this form of chronic cardiac disease and its separation from chronic rheumatic heart failure are due to the correlation of pathological and bacteriological results with physical signs, such as the presence of clubbed fingers and petechiae and the rarity of pericarditis and auricular fibrillation; this shows, if it were needed, that clinical observation is still a most important means of making advances in the science of medicine.

DISEASES OF THE VALVES OF THE HEART

Congenital heart disease. Cardiac malformations have been noted since the first treatise devoted to heart disease, Senac's *Traité de la structure du cœur, de son action et ses maladies,* published in 1749, in which a case of complete absence of the interventricular septum was recorded, the cyanosis being explained as due to admixture of venous and arterial blood, and the time of Morgagni (1761), who reported pulmonary stenosis and ascribed the cyanosis to venous stasis. Bouillaud (1835) recognized the two origins—arrest of development and foetal endocarditis; Hope (1834) believed that far the most frequent cause was a defect or premature cessation in the process of development, but it was not until 1906 that the cause of congenital heart disease was shown by Keith to be due, in the majority of cases, to an arrest of development of the bulbus cordis, and not to foetal endocarditis, as suggested by Kreysig (1817) and urged by Rokitansky. The morbid anatomy of congenital heart lesions was specially investigated by Louis, Bouillaud, Peacock (1858), Rokitansky (1875), and Maude Abbott (1908). Partial defects of the interventricular septum with freedom from cyanosis (maladie de Roger) was described by Roger (1879) and given the eponymous title by Dupré in 1891. A clinical classification according to the presence or absence of cyanosis by Bamberger (1857) was followed by much discussion about the causation of the cyanosis, and it is interesting to note that the two original views of admixture and of venous stasis, acting singly or in combination, are in the light of modern investigation the most powerful factors in the production of cardiac cyanosis (Lundsgaarde and van Slyke). Congenital heart block in association with congenital morbus cordis has been reported in sixteen cases (Maude Abbott). The liability to malignant endocarditis was pointed out in 1844 by James Paget (*vide* p. 36).

Laennec and Rokitansky believed that cyanosis was antagonistic to tuberculosis, but Peacock showed the frequency of pulmonary tuberculosis in pulmonary stenosis. The wholesale examinations during the War proved the relative longevity of persons with evidence of congenital heart disease and their comparative freedom from tuberculosis. Laennec never had an opportunity of listening with the stethoscope to a case of congenital heart disease, but assumed that useful diagnostic signs would not be thus provided. Hope (1839) recognized a superficial systolic murmur and diagnosed pulmonary stenosis and a patent interventricular septum before this was confirmed by necropsy; he also discussed the haemo-dynamics of the intra-cardiac circulation. Babington showed a specimen before the Pathological Society of London in 1847 from a patient under Thomas Addison, and mentioned that Wilkinson King during life had correctly "diagnosticated patescence of the ductus arteriosus". Bernutz also diagnosed the condition and wrote an account of it in 1849, Gerhardt (1867) investigated the physical signs, and the peculiar long murmur interested Müller and G. A. Gibson.

Mitral incompetence. Though morbid changes in the mitral valve were recognized by Morgagni (1761), the clinical features and diagnosis were first made clear by James Hope in 1832, who also seems to have been the first to realize the factor of regurgitation through the cardiac valves, and to have come to this conclusion in June 1825 in reference to human disease; this was therefore before his experimental observations in 1830 and subsequent years on the murmurs produced by rendering the valve segments incompetent. He also recognized that mitral regurgitation might be due to widening of the orifice, consequent on dilatation of the left ventricle, rendering the valves, though otherwise healthy, incapable of closing it, a view later confirmed by McDowel (1853), Stokes (1854), and Gairdner (1856). In addition he gave an intelligible account of the venous stasis caused by cardiac failure; but, as so often happens, the same idea was maturing in more minds than one, and strictly speaking Adams of Dublin in 1827 has priority over Hope in enunciating what Forget subsequently called the law of retro-dilatation of the left auricle and the right ventricle (*vide* Stokes). Before this D. Monro in 1755 had noted the association of dropsy with mitral stenosis; and William Cullen (1789) of Edinburgh, John Ferriar (1799) of Manchester, from their reasons for giving digitalis in dropsy (*vide* p. 115), seem to have associated dropsy with cardiac failure, and so prepared the way on which Corvisart (1806) travelled further to the conception of cardiac dropsy. Accentuation of the second sound over the pulmonary artery in mitral disease was pointed out by Hope (1839) and emphasized by Skoda.

Mitral stenosis, though noted in 1669 by John Mayou (1640–79), was more fully described pathologically in 1715 by Raymond de Vieussens (1641–1716), Professor of Medicine at Montpellier, who also noticed the characters of the pulse; Giambattista (1682–1771) also described it. Its clinical recognition naturally waited on the discovery of auscultation, though in 1806 Corvisart (1755–1821) insisted on the diagnostic value of the thrill. The presystolic murmur was apparently heard by Bertin in 1824, but it was not until 1843 that its importance was fully recognized by Fauvel, who must be given due credit for this correlation; he acknowledged that he obtained the word from Gendrin who coined it with some five others to indicate precisely the rhythm of the various cardiac murmurs, but does not appear to have had any knowledge of this particular murmur or its significance. James Hope (1801–41), who by vivisection established the causes of the heart sounds, described in 1832 the early diastolic murmur, once called Hope's murmur and more recently explained as due to dilatation of the pulmonary artery from high pressure and valvular incompetence, and mentioned the possibility that the auricular contraction would produce a murmur, but goes on to say that, though he had carefully looked for it, he had failed to convince himself of its existence. In 1840 his one-time colleague and subsequent rival, C. J. B. Williams (1805–89), believed a diastolic murmur in mitral obstruction to be very rare. It may seem strange that the presystolic murmur remained unaccepted for a number of years;

Canstatt in Germany in 1848 was the first authority to agree with Fauvel; in France Hérard admitted in 1853 that mitral stenosis might occasionally produce a presystolic murmur, and in 1854 Stokes mentioned the presystolic murmur but without approval. Austin Flint of New York in 1859 definitely accepted it, and in England W. H. Walshe was the first to follow suit; W. T. Gairdner in 1861, preferring to call it auricular systolic, appears to have been really responsible for its recognition in this country; this, however, was not brought about without opposition; for Ormerod (1864), A. W. Barclay (1872), W. H. Dickinson (1887), and Brockbank, though recognizing its distinctive characters and diagnostic significance, argued that it was systolic in time.

The three stages of mitral stenosis—with perfect compensation, when it is strained, and when it has completely broken down—were clearly correlated together with the physical signs by William Broadbent in 1886. The extreme irregularity of the pulse, and the change from a regular rhythm, which were noted by Stokes, were shown, after Mackenzie's polygraph work had prepared the way, by Lewis to be due to auricular fibrillation.

It is not without interest to note that pulmonary apoplexies, described and so named by Laennec (1819), appear to have been first correlated with mitral stenosis by J. A. Wilson in a paper read at this College on 22 March 1830, but only reported briefly in the *London Medical Gazette* (*vide* W. L. Dickinson), and also by Hope and Thomas Watson about the same time. Adams in 1827 described a ball clot loose in the left auricle capable of occluding the orifice, as Stokes later said, like a bullet and so causing sudden death.

The possibility of operative treatment of mitral obstruction which naturally followed the all-round advances of surgery, was voiced by Lauder Brunton (1902), investigated experimentally by Cushing and Branch (1908) and Allen (1924), and performed on man by different techniques by Cutler (1923) and by Souttar (1925).

Aortic incompetence. In 1715 Raymond de Vieussens (1641–1716) gave an account of the morbid changes and the character of the pulse in a patient with this valvular lesion, William Cooper having in 1703 described the change in the valves. The Royal College of Surgeons' Museum contains a specimen of aortic incompetence described by John Hunter. In 1829 Thomas Hodgkin (1798–1866) published a modest reference to "retroversion of the aortic valves", disclaiming any originality and saying that C. Aston Key had drawn his attention to it; Laennec and Bertin had indeed described this retroversion of the aortic valves. Hodgkin gave a good pathological and clinical account of the disease, noting the murmurs, the dilatation and hypertrophy of the heart, and the arterial pulsation, but did not anticipate Corrigan in his more complete account. Hodgkin's contribution would have been even more completely forgotten had it not been for the dutiful loyalty of Samuel Wilks and William Hale-White. In 1832 Hope described the jerking character of the pulse in cases combined with adherent pericardium and other lesions. Soon after this Dominic Corrigan (1802–80) independently published his paper "On permanent Patency of the Mouth of the Aorta, or Inadequacy of the Aortic Valves" (1832), which has perpetuated his name in Corrigan's pulse.

The important part played by syphilitic aortitis in the production of aortic incompetence has been made more obvious by the Wassermann reaction, some statistics showing that it is responsible for a majority of the cases. The syphilitic aortitis spreads to the valves, and is prone to occlude the orifices of the coronary arteries. It is significant that no other cardiac valve is prone to be involved by syphilis. The association of aortic disease and tabes was noticed long before the era of the Wassermann reaction showed how frequently syphilis was responsible for this form of valvular disease, and was probably first pointed out in 1879 by Berger and Rosenbach.

A presystolic murmur at the apex in cases of aortic incompetence and due to the normal segments of the mitral valve being rapidly floated up by the regurgitant flow from the aorta and being then set into vibration was described by Austin Flint in 1862 and again in 1886, some scepticism having been expressed about the "Austin Flint murmur," especially by Balfour of Edinburgh. Guitéras explained the presystolic murmur as due to functional mitral stenosis, especially when, from disease of the posterior aortic segment, the anterior cusp of the mitral is actively driven against the auricular stream of blood. Thayer's investigation of the incidence of Flint's murmur in cases of aortic regurgitation verified by necropsy, showed that it was present in sixty-three per cent. of cases uncomplicated by any mitral disease.

The capillary pulsation or visible ebb and flow of blood in the skin and mucous membranes known to occur in several conditions, but more especially in aortic incompetence, was first described by Quincke in 1868, Lebert in 1861 having noted it in aortic aneurysm. Brunton (1844–1916) found evidence that in the artificially made red streak there were, in addition to a wave corresponding to the pulse, another corresponding to the respirations and a third due to rhythmic pulsations at the rate of three a minute. The resources of capillary microscopy and recently of cinematographic films (Crawford) have been brought into use in order to settle the question whether the capillary pulsation is transmitted from the arterioles or is due to contraction of the capillary walls, and do not support the view that the pulsation is cardiac (Crawford and Rosenberger).

Aortic stenosis. This lesion was first noted in 1646 by Riverius (Lazare Vivière, 1589–1655) and then by Vieussens, but its clinical features were not recognized till after the advent of auscultation in the nineteenth century, and then largely due to Hope's clear account of the physical signs in 1832. Usually a disease of advanced life, cases in rare instances occur in early life; it may be a congenital abnormality due, as Keith pointed out, to arrested development of the bulbus cordis, and analogous to the much commoner lesion on the right side of the heart. Cases of this subaortic stenosis, consisting in an annular thickening of the endocardium below the aortic valves, have been ascribed to failure of the bulbus cordis to atrophy. As in other congenital lesions endocarditis is prone to supervene (*vide* p. 36). Gallavardin (1921) has described cases of aortic stenosis in early life which he ascribes to an inflammation of unknown origin occurring after birth; possibly such cases may be due to foetal endocarditis.

Tricuspid stenosis was described as a morbid lesion

by Crüwell (1765) and by Morgagni (1769) in patients observed during life and found after death to have mitral stenosis. Similar cases were reported by Corvisart (1806), Horn (1808), Allan Burns (1809), Laennec (1823), and Bertin (1824). Mitral stenosis was present in 103 out of 114 cases collected by Leudet.

Tricuspid incompetence. Dilatation of the right ventricle, like that of the left ventricle, was known to the early morbid anatomists; Lancisi ascribed the jugular pulsation observed by Galen to dilatation of the right ventricle. Adams (1827) anticipated T. Wilkinson King in recognizing the safety valve action of the tricuspid valve.

DISEASES OF THE ARTERIES

Coarctation of the aorta. This striking condition of narrowing or even obliteration of the aorta at or immediately below its isthmus, namely, the portion between the orifice of the left subclavian artery and the insertion of the ductus arteriosus, was first described in 1789 by Paris, who came upon it in the course of injecting a body for dissection; Laennec had seen three or four cases and referred to four recorded cases of obliteration, including those of Graham, John Bell, and Ashley Cooper. An early case was in a man aged ninety-two years reported by Reynaud in 1828. Peacock collected forty-six cases in 1866, and in 1903 a total of 160 was analysed by Bonnet, who divided them into (i) the infantile or developmental with usually a diffuse narrowing at the isthmus, and (ii) the adult with a sudden constriction at the site of the ductus due to post-natal cicatricial contraction.

Acute arteritis and aortitis. Though in his twenty-sixth letter Morgagni (1761) recorded a case of acute aortitis, acute arteritis did not, probably from the difficulty of distinguishing inflammation from post-mortem imbibition, and in spite of the writings of J. P. Frank (1792), Reil and Schönlein, become firmly established until Virchow recognized acute peri- and mes-aortitis. Acute inflammation of the first part of the aorta may be secondary to acute pericarditis or to malignant endocarditis of the aortic valves. Acute arteritis due to embolism of the lumen or of the vasa vasorum in bacterial endocarditis is well known since Kirkes' and Virchow's researches on embolism (*vide* p. 34). Acute aortitis, like malignant endocarditis, may supervene on previously damaged areas; it has also been found in hypoplasia of the aorta. Acute arteritis and aortitis are now known to occur in many infectious diseases; in small-pox, scarlet fever, influenza; Osler recorded it in twenty-one out of fifty-two cases of enteric fever; a special tuberculous aortitis has been described.

R   4

Arteriosclerosis. Present, as Armand Ruffer and others have shown, in the ancient Egyptians 3000 years ago, the disease, which received the name of arteriosclerosis from Lobstein in 1833 and other titles since in accordance with the various views of its causation and nature, was mentioned by William Harvey (1649) as converting portions of the aorta in noblemen into a bony tube, and was also recognized by his contemporary opponent John Riolan the younger (1577–1657), by Lancisi (1654–1720), Haller, Morgagni, Bichat, Scarpa, and others. It was first chiefly of interest as a cause of aneurysm, both arteriosclerosis and aneurysm being ascribed to syphilis or its mercurial treatment. Bertin and Bouillaud (1824) regarded the change as due to chronic inflammation, and Hope (1832), while critically debating this factor, raised that of strain and merely mentioned the opinion of others that syphilis causes arteriosclerosis. Virchow established the inflammatory nature of the process, did away with Rokitansky's hypothesis of a dyscrasic deposit from the blood, and introduced the term chronic endarteritis deformans. Though the final distinction between luetic arteritis and ordinary arteriosclerosis had to await the advent of histology, the syphilitic origin of arterial disease passed into the background at the end of the eighteenth century, to be revived about the middle of the last century. Welch, writing on aneurysm in the British Army (1876), distinguished two forms of chronic arterial disease, one causing aneurysm and in at least fifty per cent. due to syphilis, the other degenerative and not concerned in the production of aneurysm.

The study of non-syphilitic arterial disease and its relation to renal lesions was greatly stimulated and advanced by Gull and Sutton's philosophical account of arterio-capillary fibrosis in 1872 as a general change not secondary, as George Johnson contended, to renal disease, though it might produce fibrotic atrophy in the kidneys in common with other parts of the body. Gull and Sutton ascribed the morbid arterio-capillary state to a hyalin-fibroid formation, which their critics suggested might be an artifact due to the glycerine used in the preparation of the sections; whereas Johnson contended that there was a muscular hypertrophy of the arterioles, and that the obstruction was in the arteriolar, not the capillary area; it is possible that both these changes may occur, though at different stages. William Broadbent's observation that the blood pressure of renal disease is lowered by amyl nitrite points to muscular contraction rather than permanent change in the vessel walls, though he agreed with Mahomed (1879) in ascribing the peripheral resistance to toxic action on the capillary walls. Recent work points to the conclusions that the high blood pressure (i) in hyperpiesia and in chronic interstitial nephritis is due to obstruction in the arterioles ("arterial hypertonus"), and (ii) in diffuse glomerulo-nephritis depends on obstruction in the capillaries ("capillary hypertonus"). Further, not only is chronic interstitial nephritis regarded as a secondary result of a general arteriolar change, but acute glomerulo-nephritis as a result of a diffuse inflammation of the capillaries (Topfer and Weiss). In scarlet fever a rise of blood pressure and oedema have been found to occur before the appearance of renal disease (Volhard; Kylin), thus confirming Mahomed's original description of the pre-albuminuric stage in 1879. Moschowitz has recently described as pseudo-, or transient, arteriosclerosis a tightening of the radials in the course of acute glomerulo-nephritis which imitates arteriosclerosis, but disappears with recovery, and is due to raised blood pressure plus muscular hypertrophy.

Much discussion has ranged as to the inflammatory or degenerative nature of chronic arterial disease; Marchand introduced the word athero-sclerosis to take the place of arteriosclerosis and to express the view that the degenerative changes are primary and not secondary. The decrescent or involutionary (Allbutt) arterial changes in the elderly, such as Mönckeberg's sclerosis, is often instanced as a form of arteriosclerosis solely due to degeneration; but

the possible influence of past infections and toxaemias must not be lost sight of, for there is a risk of
making an artificial separation from the obviously
infective forms of arteriosclerosis, for example, after
rheumatic and typhoid fevers on which Thayer insisted, Friedländer's obliterative arteritis and the
allied thrombo-angiitis obliterans (Buerger) which
has such a racial predilection for the Jews. Thoma's
compensatory hypothesis of intimal thickening to
buttress up the arterial wall against weakness of the
media is attractive in explaining how the mechanical
strain of long-continued high blood pressure and the
resulting failure in the media caused arteriosclerosis,
and indeed is applicable to a similar sequence in
toxic degeneration of the media. The causation of the
forms of chronic arterial disease is still much discussed; that its frequency in the aged who have long
been exposed to toxic and infective factors, its
occurrence after infections, such as enteric, scarlet,
and even rheumatic fever (Klotz), and chronic toxic
conditions, such as plumbism, its association with
high blood pressure, which as Allbutt insisted is the
primary factor, and that degenerative and inflammatory changes are so often combined, are well
known. The question is which is the primary factor—
the inflammatory or the degenerative? The analogy
with syphilitic arteritis is a warning against dis-
missing inflammation as at any rate part of the

process, and in his Goulstonian Lectures Geoffrey Evans, while admitting a degenerative origin for senile arteriosclerosis, argued that diffuse hyperplastic sclerosis is due to a blood-borne bacterial toxin.

In 1839 Hope stated that arteriosclerosis, though in all probability causing deterioration of the general health, does not present any distinctly appreciative signs apart from the structural alterations. C. J. B. Williams (1840) remarked: "aortitis is scarcely known but by its anatomical characteristics". Gangrene of the extremities from arterial disease was recognized by Boerhaave, Monro, and Meckel; and intermittent claudication, originally described in the horse by H. Bouley (1831) and Goubaux (1846) was in 1858 shown to occur in man by Charcot (*vide* p. 89). Ossification of the coronary arteries was associated with angina pectoris by Edward Jenner and Parry (*vide* p. 89). The widespread—cerebral, renal, cardiac —effects of generalized arteriosclerosis were elucidated by Gull and Sutton's conception of arteriocapillary fibrosis.

Arteriosclerosis of the pulmonary artery, described by Corvisart, is mentioned by Laennec and Hope as a rarity. A case of massive dilatation with ossification on its internal surface was seen by Ambroise Paré (1510–90). Recently the recognition of a special syndrome of cyanosis, polycythaemia, dyspnoea, haemoptysis, with terminal failure of the right side of the heart—Ayerza's disease—in association with advanced sclerosis of the pulmonary artery has drawn attention to a change long known to occur in a minor degree in obstructive left-sided heart disease and pulmonary emphysema. The condition of "cardiacos negros", so named in 1901 by Ayerza of Buenos Aires and described by Arrillaga (1913), may be due to syphilis (Rogers; Warthin) or to arteriosclerosis of other origin (Clarke, Coombs, Hadfield, and Todd). It is closely allied to the Vaquez-Osler syndrome.

Syphilitic arteritis. The syphilitic factor of arterial disease, which had been current in the seventeenth and eighteenth centuries, was revived in the middle of the last century by Dittrich (1849), Virchow, Steenberg (1860), Wilks (1863), and in 1868 the first histological account of syphilitic arteritis was given by Clifford Allbutt, but Heubner's description in 1874, being more easily accessible, attracted attention; in 1877 Thomas Barlow reported its occurrence in congenital lues. Mesaortitis, obliterative endarteritis of the vasa vasorum, and the presence of the *Spironema pallidum* in the media (Reuter; Schmorl; Benda; Warthin) were subsequently established. Syphilitic aortitis has been found histologically in more than half the patients with a positive Wassermann reaction.

Aneurysm. Among the diseases of the cardio-
vascular system aneurysm stands out as having by
its obvious features forced due recognition long
before the circulation was discovered, thus con-
trasting with cardiac disease which up to the
eighteenth century was thought not to occur.
Antyllos (A.D. 55–118) operated upon it, and Galen
(A.D. 130–200) described two forms—the traumatic
and spontaneous. The traumatic and superficial
aneurysm was that mainly seen until syphilis became
widespread after the return in 1493 of Columbus
from the New World and the occupation of Naples
by the army of Charles VIII in 1495; there was then
what has been called an unprecedented occurrence
of aortic aneurysm. The association with syphilis did
not escape Fernelius who in 1542 first recognized
internal aneurysms, Vesalius who about 1557
diagnosed both thoracic and abdominal aneurysms,
and Ambroise Paré (1582) who incriminated mercurial treatment as a cause of aneurysm. The luetic
origin of aneurysm, though accepted by Lancisi
(1728) and Morgagni (1761), waned; Matthew
Baillie did not mention it in 1789 or later; but it was
revived on good grounds in the middle of the last
century by Crisp (1847), Myers (1871), Welch (1875)
in this country, and by many foreign authors. Early
in this century the Wassermann reaction (1906)
facilitated the detection of clinically latent syphilis,

and early changes in and around the vasa vasorum of the aorta (mesaortitis, Heller) and the presence there of the *Spironema pallidum* (Schaudinn and Hoffmann, 1905) fully established the paramount importance of syphilis in the etiological relationship of aneurysm.

Joseph Hodgson (1788–1869) in 1815 described, as distinct from aneurysm, "praeternatural dilatation of the arteries" which has been called Hodgson's or Hodgson-Welch disease and is now assumed to be syphilitic; but examination of his text and plates shows that it is a fusiform dilatation or aneurysm, which when in the vicinity of the aortic valves stretches the ring and makes them incompetent. His account was written some years before aortic regurgitation was described by Hodgkin (1829) and Corrigan (1832).

In aneurysm, particularly intrathoracic, though syphilis is in the vast number of instances the important underlying factor, the influence of strain as an immediate exciting cause must not be overlooked; further, in some instances, luetic infection is not concerned: in old people dissecting aneurysms and abdominal aneurysms may be due to ordinary arteriosclerosis. Hypoplasia of the arterial system has been found to be a cause of aneurysm (W. L. Dickinson), and acute multiple aneurysms are due to malignant endocarditis.

Embolic aneurysms were first described by W. S. Church in 1870; in 1873 Ponfick published an account of cases in a more accessible journal. The embolic aneurysm, at first considered to be due to injury, for example by a calcified spicule, and to occur specially in ill-supported vessels, such as the mesenteric and those at the base of the brain, has long been recognized as in the vast majority of instances mycotic-embolic and due to infection, as in malignant or subacute bacterial endocarditis. In addition to obvious embolism of the lumen of the artery it has been thought that embolism of the vasa vasorum may be responsible. Periarteritis nodosa was described by Kussmaul and Maier in 1866.

Dissecting aneurysm, as found in the body of George II, was described in 1760 by Frank Nicholls (1699–1778), whose experiments had shown that the two inner coats of arteries can be ruptured while the external coat remains intact. The name "dissecting" was first used by Maunoir in 1802; Laennec gave a careful description of a case, and Peacock, Boström, and Adami made collections of the known cases. It may result from sharp-cut ruptures of the internal coats at the commencement of the aorta, or be due to ordinary atheromatous ulceration. Dissecting aneurysm of the heart is mentioned on p. 22.

The occurrence of *arterio-venous aneurysm* as the result of clumsy venesection was clearly shown by

William Hunter (1757), thus confirming what Galen, Aetius, and Guillemeau (1594) had long before noticed. The picture produced by arterio-venous aneurysm, which has been regarded as that of aortic incompetence or of myocardial failure with well-marked hepatic pulsation and enlargement of both ventricles but not of the auricles, has been investigated clinically and experimentally by Hoover and Beams; they conclude that the ventricular enlargement is compensatory in order to deal with the increased minute volume flow, and that the hepatic pulsation is due to the increased venous pressure. Cure of the arterio-venous aneurysm is followed by the disappearance of the cardiac, hepatic and blood pressure changes.

Abdominal aneurysm, first diagnosed clinically by Vesalius, was recorded post-mortem by his contemporaries Falloppius and Ballonius. Matthew Baillie distinguished simple dynamic pulsation from aneurysm of the abdominal aorta.

Harvey in the *De Motu Cordis* commented on the difference in the pulse on the two sides. MacDonnell in 1850 and W. H. Walshe (1812–92) in 1853 drew attention to the condition of the pupil in aortic aneurysm; in 1854 Stokes recognized laryngeal paralysis, and the law that the abductor fibres suffer first was established by F. Semon (1898). Tracheal tugging was first, and in remarkably brief terms, described by W. S. Oliver in 1878. In 1896, within a short time of Roentgen's discovery in 1895, X-rays were employed in the diagnosis of cardiac enlargement (Macintyre).

Treatment. Valsalva's method, as recorded and practised by Albertini (1748) and by Morgagni (1761), consisted in small bleedings repeated weekly combined with rest and low diet, and was in vogue during the eighteenth century. Tufnell's treatment (1874) consisted in a much-restricted intake of food and fluid and of complete rest. Iodide of potassium[1] was extensively used, first by Nelaton (1859), Bouillaud, Chuckerbutty (1862), on the assumption that it increased the coagulating power of the blood, and later especially by W. Roberts and G. W. Balfour. Lancereaux (1897) advocated the subcutaneous injection of a solution of gelatine to promote coagulation in the sac; but the occurrence of tetanus in a few cases acted as a deterrent in this country.

William Murray employed compression for abdominal aneurysm in 1864. Ligature of the aorta has been uniformly fatal. Moore's method of introducing wire into the aneurysm sac (1864) to induce

[1] Iodide of potassium appears to have been first used in tertiary syphilis in 1831 by R. Williams (*vide* H. Marsh, *St Barth. Hosp. Rep.* 1900, xxxvi, 6); W. Wallace of Dublin (*Lancet*, 1836, ii, 5) has also been credited with this advance.

coagulation has been modified in various ways, for example by D'Arcy Power and Colt. Corradi practised electrolysis by means of the wire, and this again was improved by Finney and Hunner. Macewen scraped the inside of the sac by a needle inserted into the aneurysm.

REFERENCES

I

GASKELL, W. H. *Journ. Physiol.* 1883, IV, 43.
KEITH, A. and FLACK, M. *Journ. Anat. and Physiol.* 1907, XLI, 172.
KENT, A. F. S. *Journ. Physiol.* 1893, XIV, 233.
TAWARA, S. Das Reizleitungsystem des Säugetierherzens. Jena, 1906.

Capillaries:

BROWNE, T. Works. Edited by S. Wilkin. 1836. Vol. I, pp. 356, 362, 365.
CLARK, E. R. and CLARK, E. L. *Am. Journ. Anat.* Baltimore, 1925, XXXV, 239.
DALE, H. H. *Bull. Johns Hopkins Hosp.* Baltimore, 1919, XXXI, 257.
DALE and LAIDLAW. *Journ. Physiol.* 1918–19, LII, 351.
DALE and RICHARDS. *Ibid.* 1918–19, LII, 110.
HOOKER, D. R. *Physiological Reviews,* Baltimore, 1921, I, 112.
INCHLEY, O. *Journ. Physiol.* Cambridge, 1926, LXI, 282.
KROGH, A. Anatomy and Physiology of the Capillaries. New Haven, 1922.
LEWIS, T. The Blood Vessels of the Human Skin and their Responses. 1927.
LOMBARD, W. D. *Am. Journ. Physiol.* 1912, XXIX, 335.
LUCIANI, L. Human Physiology. English ed. 1911. Vol. I, p. 172.
ROUGET, C. *Compt. rend. Acad. sc.* Paris, 1873, LXXIX, 559.
—— *Arch. de physiol. norm. et path.* 1873, V, 603.
ROY, C. S. and BROWN, G. *Journ. Physiol.* Cambridge, 1879, II, 323.
VIMTRUP, B. *Ztschr. ges. Anat.* 1922, LXV, 150.
YOUNG, T. Croonian Lecture, Roy. Soc. 1808.

62 ANATOMICO-CLINICAL HISTORY

Diseases of the Pericardium:

ALLBUTT, T. C. *Lancet*, 1869, i, 807.

ANDRAL, G. *Clinique médicale*, 1829, I, 55.

BERTIN, R. J. Traité des maladies du cœur et des gros vaisseaux. Rédigé par J. Bouillaud. 1824. P. 239.

BRIGHT, R. *Med.-Chir. Trans.* 1839, XXII, 10.

BROADBENT, J. Adherent Pericardium. London, 1895.

BROADBENT, W. *Trans. Path. Soc. Lond.* 1882, XXXIII, 78.

COLLIN, V. Des diverses méthodes d'exploration de la poitrine. Paris, 1824. P. 115.

DOUGLAS, J. S. C. *Med. Chron.* Manchester, 1906–7, s. 4, XII, 207.

GILBERT et GARNIER. *Compt. rend. Soc. biol.* Paris, 1898, L, 48.

HEIDEMANN. *Berlin. klin. Wchnschr.* 1897, XXXIV, 92.

HOPE, J. A Treatise on Diseases of the Heart and Great Vessels. Ed. 3. 1839. P. 191.

KUSSMAUL, A. *Berlin. klin. Wchnschr.* 1873, I, 433.

PICK, F. *Ztschr. f. klin. Med.* 1896, XXIX, 385.

SCHWARZ, G. *Wien. klin. Wchnschr.* 1910, XXIII, 1850.

TAYLOR, F. *Brit. Med. Journ.* 1900, II, 1698.

TROUSSEAU, A. Lectures on Clinical Medicine. New Sydenham Soc. 1870. Vol. III, p. 374.

TROUSSEAU et LASÈGUE. *Arch. gén. de méd.* Paris, 1854, s. 5, IV, 513.

WEST, S. *Med.-Chir. Trans.* 1883, LXVI, 235.

WILKS, S. *Guy's Hosp. Rep.* 1871, s. 3, XVI, 196.

WILLIAMS, C. J. B. Pathology and Diagnosis of Diseases of the Chest. 1840. P. 239.

Diseases of the Myocardium:

BURNS, A. Observations on some of the most important Diseases of the Heart. 1809. P. 163.

STOKES, W. Diseases of the Heart and Aorta. 1854. P. 131.

Fatty Degeneration:

CHEYNE, J. *Dublin Hosp. Rep.* 1816, II, 217.

COOMBE, J. G. and KELLIE, G. *Trans. Med.-Chir. Soc. Edin.* 1824, I, 194.

DICKINSON, W. H. *Trans. Path. Soc. London*, 1863, XIV, 141.

ORMEROD, E. L. *London Med. Gaz.* 1849, IX, 739.

PAGET, J. *Ibid.* 1847, V, 143.

QUAIN, R. *Med.-Chir. Trans.* 1850, s. 2, XV, 121–196.

STOKES, W. Diseases of the Heart and Aorta. 1854. P. 324.
WILSON, L. B. *Trans. Assoc. Am. Phys.* Phila. 1923, XXXVIII, 144.

Fibroid Disease and Cardiac Aneurysm:

BAILLIE, M. The Morbid Anatomy of some of the most important Parts of the Human Body. 1818. P. 24.
BRESCHET. Répertoire d'anatomie et de physiologie path. 1827. Vol. III, p. 181.
FAGGE, C. H. *Trans. Path. Soc. Lond.* 1874, XXV, 64.
GAIRDNER, W. T. *Month. Journ. Med. Sc.* Edin. and London, 1854, XIX, 79.
HEKTOEN, L. *Trans. Assoc. Am. Phys.* Phila. 1901, XVI, 127.
HUBER, K. *Virchows Arch.* 1882, LXXXIX, 236.
LEGG, J. W. Some Account of Cardiac Aneurysms (Bradshaw Lecture, 1883). 8vo. London, 1884.
QUAIN, R. *Trans. Path. Soc. Lond.* 1850, III, 282.
STEVEN, J. L. *Lancet*, London, 1887, ii, 1153.
THURNAM, J. *Med.-Chir. Trans.* 1838, XXI, 187.
TURNER, F. C. *Trans. Internat. Congr. Med.* London, 1881, I, 427.
VESTBERG, A. *Nord. Med. Ark.* 1897, n. F., VIII, Heft 5.
WEIGERT, C. *Virchows Arch.* 1880, LXXIX, 390.
WILKS, S. *Trans. Path. Soc. Lond.* 1857, VIII, 150.

Mechanical Strain:

ADAMI, J. G. *Interstate Med. Journ.* 1911, XVIII, 601.
ALLBUTT, T. C. *St George's Hosp. Rep.* 1870, V, 23.
—— System of Medicine, 1898, V, 841; 1909, VI, 193.
ANDRAL, G. *Clinique médicale*, Paris, 1830, III, 530.
BRIGHT, R. Medical Reports. 1827. P. 23. *Guy's Hosp. Rep.* 1836, I, 9.
COLLIER, W. *Trans. Med. Soc. Lond.* 1893, XVI, 64.
DA COSTA, J. M. *Am. Journ. Med. Sc.* Phila. 1871, LXI, 1.
HOPE, J. A Treatise on the Diseases of the Heart and Great Vessels. Ed. 3. 1839. P. 245.
LEWIS, T. Med. Research Committee: Special Rep. Series, No. 8. 1917.
MORGAN, J. E. University Oars. 1873. P. 29.
MYERS, A. B. R. Etiology and Prevalence of Diseases of the Heart among Soldiers. London, 1870.
ROY, C. S. and ADAMI, J. G. *Brit. Med. Journ.* 1888, ii, 1321.
TRAUBE, L. *Berlin. klin. Wchnschr.* 1872, IX, 223.

Rheumatic Myocarditis:

Aschoff, L. *Verhandl. d. deutsch. path. Gesellsch.* 1905, VIII, 46.
Barlow, T. and Warner, F. *Trans. Internat. Congress,* London, 1881, IV, 116.
Coombs, C. *Quart. Journ. Med.* Oxford, 1908–9, II, 26.
Fagge, C. H. Principles and Practice of Medicine. 1886. Vol. II, p. 29.
Hillier, T. *Med. Times and Gaz.* 1863, II, 142.
Hope, J. A Treatise on Diseases of the Heart and Great Vessels. Ed. 3. 1839. P. 247.
Lees, D. B. *Med.-Chir. Trans.* 1898, LXXXI, 401.
Lees and Poynton. *Ibid.* 1898, LXXXI, 419.
Poynton, F. J. *Ibid.* 1899, LXXXII, 355.
Sansom, A. E. *Internat. Clinics,* Phila. 1894, s. 4, I, 1.
Steell, G. *Med. Chron.* Manchester, 1896–7, N.S. VI, 321.
Wilks, S. Lectures on Pathological Anatomy. Ed. '3. 1889. P. 125.

Alcoholic Heart:

Allbutt, T. C. *Practitioner,* 1902, LXVIII, 11.
Bauer und Bollinger. Festschrift f. Pettenkofer. München, 1893.
Steell, G. *Med. Chron.* Manchester, 1893, XVIII, 1.

Tumours of the Myocardium:

Beck and Thatcher. *Arch. Int. Med.* Chicago, 1925, XXXVI, 830.
Billard. Traité des maladies des enfants nouveau-nés et à la mamelle. Paris, 1828.
Hope, J. A Treatise on Diseases of the Heart and Great Vessels. Ed. 3. 1839. P. 355.
Howland, J. Contributions to Medical and Biological Research Dedicated to Sir W. Osler. 1919. Vol. I, p. 582.
Perlstein, I. *Am. Journ. Med. Sc.* Phila. 1918, CLVI, 214.
Virchow, R. *Berlin. klin. Wchnschr.* 1896, XXXIII, 679.
Walshe, W. H. Treatise on Diseases of the Heart and Great Vessels. 1862. P. 358.
Wolbach, S. B. *Journ. Med. Res.* Boston, 1907, XVI, 495.

Hydatids:

DAVAINE. Traité des entozoaires. 1860.
DÉVÉ, F. *Algérie méd.* 1928, mai.
PEACOCK, T. B. System of Medicine (Russell Reynolds). 1877. Vol. IV, p. 172.
TROTTER, T. Medical and Chemical Essays. 1795. P. 123.

Acute Endocarditis:

BAILLIE, M. The Morbid Anatomy of the Human Body. Ed. 2. 1797. Ed. 5. 1818. P. 51.
BILLINGS, F. Focal Infections. New York, 1906.
BLAINCOURT, I. B. Essai sur le salicine. Paris, 1830.
BOUILLAUD, J. B. Nouvelles recherches sur la rhumatisme articulaire. Paris, 1836.
DUNDAS, D. *Med.-Chir. Trans.* 1809, I, 37.
ELLIOTSON, J. *Lancet*, London, 1831, i, 554.
FAGGE, C. H. Principles and Practice of Medicine. 1886. Vol. II, p. 539.
FULLER, H. W. On Rheumatism, Rheumatic Gout and Sciatica. 1860.
GULL and SUTTON. *Med.-Chir. Trans.* 1869, LII, 43.
HOPE, J. A Treatise on Diseases of the Heart and Great Vessels. 1832.
HUNTER, W. *Brit. Med. Journ.* 1900, ii, 215.
JACOBS, H. B. Contributions to Medical and Biological Research dedicated to Sir William Osler. 1919. Vol. II, p. 745 (containing a letter from Jenner to C. H. Parry, in the possession of Dr Jacobs).
KREYSIG. Krankheiten des Herzens. 1814–17.
LATHAM, P. M. *London Med. Gaz.* 1828–9, III, 209, 214.
—— Lectures on Subjects connected with Clinical Medicine comprising Diseases of the Heart. 1845. P. 101.
LEES, D. B. Treatment of Some Acute Visceral Inflammations. 1904.
MACLAGAN, T. J. *Lancet*, London, 1876, i, 342, 910.
POYNTON, F. J. and PAINE, A. *Ibid.* 1900, ii, 861, 932.
REES, O. On the Treatment of Rheumatic Diseases by Lemon Juice. 1849.
SIBSON, F. System of Medicine (Russell Reynolds). 1877. Vol. IV, p. 527.

WELLS, W. C. *Trans. Soc. Improvement of Med. and Chirurg. Know-ledge*, 1812, III, 373.

Malignant Endocarditis :

ABBOTT, M. E. *Ann. Clin. Med.* 1925, IV, 189.
BAEHR, G. *Journ. Exper. Med.* 1912, XV, 330.
BARLOW and REES. *Guy's Hosp. Rep.* 1843, N.S. I, 227.
BOUILLAUD, J. B. Traité clinique des maladies du cœur. 1841. Vol. II, p. 308.
CHARCOT et VULPIAN. *Mém. Soc. biol.* Paris, 1861, 3 s., III, 205.
CORVISART, J. N. Essai sur les maladies et les lésions organiques du cœur. Paris, 1806.
—— Treatise on Diseases of the Heart and Great Vessels, trans-lated by C. H. Hebb. 1813. P. 195.
GARROD, A. E. *Trans. Path. Soc. Lond.* 1897, XLVIII, 42.
HODGSON, J. A Treatise on Diseases of the Arteries and Veins. London, 1815. Plate I, Fig. 7.
HORDER, T. *Quart. Journ. Med.* Oxford, 1908–9, II, 289.
JACCOUD. Clinique de la Pitié. 1885–6.
KIRKES, W. S. *Med.-Chir. Trans.* 1852, XXXV, 281.
LEWIS and GRANT. *Heart*, London, 1923, X, 21.
LIBMAN, E. *Am. Journ. Med. Sc.* Phila. 1910, CXL, 516.
—— *Trans. XVII Internat. Congress Med.* London, 1913, Sect. Med. 196.
ORMEROD, E. L. *London Med. Gaz.* 1851, N.S. XII, 617, 619, 677.
OSLER, W. *Brit. Med. Journ.* 1885, i, 467, 522, 577.
—— *Trans. Assoc. Am. Phys.* Phila. 1886, I, 185.
—— *Quart. Journ. Med.* Oxford, 1908–9, II, 219.
PAGET, J. *Med.-Chir. Trans.* 1844, XXVII, 162.
POYNTON, F. J. and PAINE, A. Researches on Rheumatism. 1913.
SCHOTTMÜLLER. *München. med. Wchnschr.* 1910, LVII, i, 617.
THAYER, W. S. *Johns Hopkins Hosp. Rep.* Baltimore, 1926, XXII, Fasc. i, 185.
THAYER and BLUMER. *Arch. de méd. expér. et d'anat. path.* Paris, 1895, VII, 701.
WILKS, S. *Guy's Hosp. Rep.* 1870, s. 3, XV, 29.

Congenital Heart Disease :

ABBOTT, M. E. Modern Medicine (Osler and McCrae). 1908. Vol. IV, p. 323.

BABINGTON, B. G. *Trans. Path. Soc. Lond.* 1847, I, 55.

BERNUTZ. *Arch. gén. de méd.* Paris, 1849, XX, 415.

BOUILLAUD, J. B. Traité clinique des maladies du cœur. Paris, 1835. Tome II, p. 544.

DUPRÉ. *Bull. Soc. anat.* Paris, 1891, s. 5, V, 404.

GIBSON, G. A. Diseases of the Heart and Aorta. 1898. P. 303.

HOPE, J. Principles and Illustrations of Morbid Anatomy. 1834. P. 96.

—— A Treatise on the Diseases of the Heart and Great Vessels. Ed. 3. 1839. P. 490.

KEITH, A. Studies in Pathology, Aberdeen Quatercentenary Celebration. 1906. P. 55.

LUNDSGAARDE and VAN SLYKE. *Medicine*, 1923, II, 1.

PEACOCK, T. B. Malformations of the Human Heart. 1858.

ROGER, H. *Bull. Acad. de méd.* Paris, 1879, s. 2, VIII, 1074.

ROKITANSKY, C. Defekte der Scheidewände des Herzens. Wien, 1875.

Mitral Incompetence:

ADAMS, R. *Dublin Hosp. Rep.* 1827, IV, 422.

GAIRDNER, W. T. *Edin. Med. Journ.* 1856, II, 55.

HOPE, J. A Treatise on the Diseases of the Heart and Great Vessels. London, 1832.

—— *Ibid.* Ed. 3. 1839. P. 69.

McDOWEL. *Dublin Journ. Med. Sc.* 1853, XVI, 76.

MONRO, D. Essay on the Dropsy and its different Species. London, 1755. P. 17. (Quoted by Comry, *Brit. Med. Journ.* 1928, ii, 230.)

SKODA, J. Abhandlung über Percussion und Auskultation. Wien, 1850.

STOKES, W. Diseases of the Heart and Aorta. 1854. Pp. 191, 271.

Mitral Stenosis:

ALLEN, D. S. *Arch. Surg.* 1924, VIII, 317.

BARCLAY, A. W. *Lancet*, London, 1872, i, 283.

BERTIN, R. J. Traité des maladies du cœur. Paris, 1824. Pp. 176, 186.

BROADBENT, W. *Am. Journ. Med. Sc.* Phila. 1886, XCI, 57.

BROCKBANK, E. M. *Brit. Med. Journ.* 1909, ii, 509, 1579.

BRUNTON, T. L. *Lancet*, London, 1902, i, 352.

CORVISART, J. N. Essai sur les maladies et les lésions organiques du cœur. Paris, 1806. P. 236.

CUSHING and BRANCH. *Journ. Med. Res.* Boston, 1908, XVII, 471.
CUTLER and LEVINE. *Boston Med. and Surg. Journ.* 1923, CLXXXVIII, 1023.
DICKINSON, W. H. *Lancet,* London, 1887, ii, 650; 1889, ii, 779.
DICKINSON, W. L. *St George's Hosp. Gaz.* 1896, IV, 161.
FAGGE, C. H. *Guy's Hosp. Rep.* 1874, s. 3, XIX, 199 (History).
FAUVEL, A. *Arch. gén. de méd.* Paris, 1843, s. 4, I, 1.
FLINT, A. Practical Treatise on the Diagnosis, Pathology, and Treatment of Diseases of the Heart. Phila. 1859.
GAIRDNER, W. T. *Edin. Med. Journ.* 1861–2, VII, 438.
—— Clinical Medicine. 1862. P. 575.
GENDRIN. Leçons sur les maladies du cœur. Paris, 1841. Tome I, p. III.
HÉRARD. *Arch. gén. de méd.* Paris, 1853, s. 5, II, 543.
HOPE, J. A Treatise on Diseases of the Heart and Great Vessels. Ed. 3. 1839. P. 79.
ORMEROD, E. L. *Med. Times and Gaz.* 1864, II, 154.
SOUTTAR, H. S. *Brit. Med. Journ.* 1925, ii, 603.
STOKES, W. Diseases of the Heart and Aorta. 1854. P. 181.
WALSHE, W. H. Practical Treatise on Diseases of the Heart. Ed. 3. 1862. Pp. 104, 372.
WILLIAMS, C. J. B. The Pathology and Diagnosis of Diseases of the Chest. 1840. P. 273.

Aortic Incompetence:

BALFOUR, G. W. Diseases of the Heart and Aorta. Ed. 2. 1882. Pp. 116, 165.
BERGER und ROSENBACH. *Berlin. klin. Wchnschr.* 1879, XVI, 402.
BERTIN, R. J. Traité des maladies du cœur et des gros vaisseaux. 1824. P. 216.
BRUNTON, T. L. *Journ. Physiol.* Cambridge, 1884, V, 14.
CORRIGAN, D. *Edin. Med. and Surg. Journ.* 1832, X, 225.
CRAWFORD, J. H. and ROSENBERGER, H. *Journ. Clin. Investig.* 1926, II, 343, 351; 1927, IV, 307.
FLINT, A. *Am. Journ. Med. Sc.* Phila. 1862, XLIV, 29; 1886, XCI, 35.
GUITÉRAS, J. *Trans. Assoc. Am. Phys.* Phila. 1887, II, 27.
HALE-WHITE, W. *Guy's Hosp. Rep.* 1924, LXXIV, 117.
HODGKIN, T. *London Med. Gaz.* 1829, III, 433.
HOPE, J. A Treatise on Diseases of the Heart and Great Vessels. London, 1832. P. 434.

HUNTER, J. Treatise on the Blood. 1794.

LEBERT. Virchows Handb. d. sp. Path. u. Therap. 1861. Bd. v, Abt. ii, s. 20.

QUINCKE, H. *Berlin. klin. Wchnschr.* 1868, v, 357.

THAYER, W. S. *Trans. Assoc. Am. Phys.* Phila. 1901, XVI, 393.

VIEUSSENS, R. Traité nouveau de la structure et des causes des mouvements du cœur. Toulouse, 1715.

WILKS, S. *Guy's Hosp. Rep.* 1871, s. 3, XVI, 211; 1878, s. 3, XXIII, 65.

Aortic Stenosis:

GALLIVARDIN, L. *Presse méd.* Paris, 1921, XLII, 23.

HOPE, J. A Treatise on the Diseases of the Heart and Great Vessels. London, 1832.

KEITH, A. Quatercentenary Studies in Pathology. Aberdeen, 1906. P. 57.

RIVERIUS. Opera Medica Universa. Frankfort, 1674. P. 638. (Quoted by G. A. Gibson, Diseases of the Heart and Aorta. 1898. P. 473.)

Tricuspid Stenosis:

BERTIN. Traité des maladies du cœur et des gros vaisseaux. Paris, 1824. P. 190.

BURNS, A. Observations on some of the most frequent and important Diseases of the Heart. Edinburgh, 1809. P. 30.

CORVISART, J. N. Essai sur les maladies et les lésions organiques du cœur et des gros vaisseaux. Paris, 1806.

CRÜWELL. De Corde et Vasorum osteogenesi in quadragenario observ. Halae, 1765.

HORN. *Arch. f. prakt. Med.* 1808, IV, 296.

LEUDET. Thèse de Paris. 1888.

Tricuspid Incompetence:

ADAMS, R. *Dublin Hosp. Rep.* 1827, IV, 436.

KING, T. W. *Guy's Hosp. Rep.* 1837, II, 132.

Coarctation of the Aorta:

BONNET, L. M. *Rev. de méd.* Paris, 1903, XXIII, 108.

LAENNEC. Mediate Auscultation. Forbes' Eng. transl. Ed. 3. 1832. P. 686.

PARIS. *Journ. de chir. de Desault*, Paris, 1789, II, 107.

REYNAUD. *Journ. hebd. de méd.* Paris, 1828, I, 161.

Acute Arteritis and Aortitis:

FRANK, J. P. Curandis hominum Morbis. 1792.
VIRCHOW, R. *Virchows Arch.* 1847, I, 272.

Arteriosclerosis:

ANDREWES, F. W. Report of the Medical Officer of the Local
    Government Board. Appendix I. 1911–12.
ARRILLAGA, F. C. Cardiacos Negros. Buenos Aires, 1913.
BROADBENT, W. The Pulse. 1890.
BUERGER, L. The Circulatory Disturbances of the Extremities.
    1924.
CLARKE, COOMBS, HADFIELD and TODD. *Quart. Journ. Med.*
    Oxford, 1927–8, XXI, 51.
CORVISART, J. N. Essai sur les maladies et les lésions organiques
    du cœur. 1911, p. 428.
EVANS, G. *Brit. Med. Journ.* 1923, i, 550.
GULL and SUTTON. *Med.-Chir. Trans.* 1872, LV, 273.
HARVEY, W. Second Disquisition to John Riolan, Jun. Willis'
    transl. of the Works of W. Harvey. Sydenham Soc. 1847.
    P. 112.
HOPE, J. A Treatise on the Diseases of the Heart and Great
    Vessels. London, 3rd edit. 1839.
JOHNSON, G. *Med.-Chir. Trans.* 1873, LVI, 276.
KLOTZ, O. University of Toronto, Pathological Series, No. 7.
    1926. P. 44.
LOBSTEIN. Traité d'anat. path. 1833.
MAHOMED, F. A. *Guy's Hosp. Rep.* 1879, s. 3, XXIV, 363.
MARCHAND, L. Verhandl. d. Congr. f. inn. Med. 1904. P. 21.
MOSCHOWITZ, E. *Journ. Am. Med. Assoc.* Chicago, 1928, XC, 1526.
ROGERS, L. *Quart. Journ. Med.* Oxford, 1908–9, II, 1.
RUFFER, M. A. *Journ. Path. and Bacteriol.* Cambridge, 1911, XV, 453.
THAYER, W. S. *Am. Journ. Med. Sc.* Phila. 1904, CXXVII, 391.
THAYER and BRUSH. *Journ. Am. Med. Assoc.* Chicago, 1904, XLIII,
    726.
THOMA, R. Textbook of General Pathology, transl. by A. Bruce.
VIRCHOW, R. *Virchows Arch.* 1847, I, 272.
WARTHIN, A. S. Contributions to Med. and Biolog. Sc. Dedicated
    to Sir W. Osler. 1919. Vol. II, p. 1042.
WELCH, F. H. *Med.-Chir. Trans.* 1876, LIX, 59.

WILLIAMS, C. J. B. Pathology and Diagnosis of Diseases of the Chest. 1840. P. 282.

Syphilitic Arteritis:

ALLBUTT, T. C. *St George's Hosp. Rep.* 1868. III, 56.
BARLOW, T. *Trans. Path. Soc.* London, 1877, XXVIII, 287.
HEUBNER. Die luetische Erkrankungen d. Hirnarterien. 1874.
VIRCHOW, R. Krankhaften Geschwulste, 1864–5, II, p. 444.

Aneurysm:

ADAMI, J. G. *Montreal Med. Journ.* 1896, XXIV, 945.
BALFOUR, G. W. Clinical Lectures on Diseases of the Heart and Aorta. Ed. 2. 1882. P. 406. (For history of potassium iodide in aneurysm.)
BOSTRÖM. *Deutsches Arch. f. klin. Med.* 1888, XLII, 1.
CHUCKERBUTTY, S. G. *Brit. Med. Journ.* 1862, ii, 61.
CHURCH, W. S. *St Barth. Hosp. Rep.* 1870, VI, 99.
D'ARCY POWER and COLT. *Med.-Chir. Trans.* 1903, LXXXVI, 363.
DICKINSON, W. L. *Trans. Path. Soc.* London, 1894, XLV, 52; 1898, XLIX, 48.
FINNEY and HUNNER. *Bull. Johns Hopkins Hosp.* Baltimore, 1900, XI, 263.
HELLER. *Verhandl. deutsch. path. Gesellsch.* 1900, II, 346.
HODGSON, J. A Treatise on Diseases of Arteries and Veins. London, 1815.
HOOVER, C. F. and BEAMS, A. J. *Trans. Assoc. Am. Phys.* Phila. 1923, XXXVIII, 6.
KUSSMAUL, A. und MAIER, R. *Deutsches Arch. f. klin. Med.* 1866, I, 484.
LANCEREAUX, E. *Bull. Acad. de méd.* Paris, 1897, XXXVII, 784.
MACEWEN, W. *Brit. Med. Journ.* 1890, ii, 1107.
MACINTYRE, J. *Lancet,* London, 1896, i, 1455.
MOORE, C. H. *Med.-Chir. Trans.* 1864, XLVII, 129.
MURRAY, W. *Ibid.* 1864, XLVII, 187.
NICHOLLS, F. *Phil. Trans.* 1760, XXXV, 443.
OLIVER, W. S. *Lancet,* London, 1878, ii, 406.
PEACOCK, T. B. *Trans. Path. Soc.* London, 1863, XIV, 87. (Collected eighty cases.)
SEMON, F. *Brit. Med. Journ.* 1898, i, 1.
STOKES, W. Diseases of the Heart and Aorta. 1854. P. 569.
TUFNELL, J. *Med.-Chir. Trans.* 1874, LVII, 83.

II

Unaided Clinical Observation

UNDER the heading of unaided clinical observation the use of the stethoscope may perhaps be included, as it is artificial to separate the employment of this instrument of precision from that of direct auscultation. In this section the history also is outlined of some cardiac disorders—dyspnoea, angina pectoris, coronary thrombosis, the Stokes-Adams syndrome, exophthalmic goitre—which give rise to characteristic clinical pictures. As would naturally be anticipated the history of cardiac diagnosis shows that in the main recognition and correlation of symptoms came first and the invention of physical methods of examination later. Albertini (1672–1733) of Bologna laid stress on palpitation and dyspnoea as evidence of cardiac disease, and ascribed the latter to venous stasis in the lungs. He also made use of palpation, which was little employed before his time or indeed for a hundred years after, until Corvisart revived it and drew attention to thrills. By his authoritative position Corvisart was able to rescue the neglected observations of his predecessors from oblivion, thus resembling Samuel Wilks in our day. He considered that organic heart disease was second in frequency only to pulmonary tuberculosis, and that eventually it was invariably fatal. In the middle of the last century Stokes of Dublin, Gairdner of Edinburgh and Glasgow, and Walshe of London were prominent in clinical cardiology. Gairdner's elucidation of the significance of cardiac murmurs was assisted by his graphic representation of their time relations. In the last quarter of the nineteenth century William Broadbent was prominent as a clinical observer.

Percussion was described by Leopold Auenbrugger (1722–1809) of Vienna in a pamphlet of twenty-two pages *Inventum novum ex Percussione Thoracis humani, ut Signo abstrusos interni pectoris Morbos detegendi* in 1761, the year in which Morgagni's great work on morbid anatomy, *De Sedibus et Causis Morborum*, appeared, and so should have been a means of correlating physical signs with gross structural changes. But though praised as worthy of all attention by his senior contemporary Albrecht von Haller of Berne, and translated into French by Rozière de la Chassagne and published in Paris in 1770, the conservatism responsible for opposition to Harvey's discovery delayed the acceptance of Auenbrugger's percussion. It was thus long before its time and did not receive any recognition until in 1808, the year before the author's death, J. N. Corvisart translated it into French for the second time, and naturally made much use of it in diagnosis, but little of auscultation, for the classical work of his pupil appeared two years only before his death. It is interesting to note that Laennec's last work as one of the Editors of the *Journal de médecine* was a review of Corvisart's translation of the *Inventum novum*. Percussion did not become generally adopted until later combined with auscultation, and was comparatively unknown in this country until the first English translation of the monograph was made in 1824 by Sir John Forbes, who in 1821 had translated Laennec's *Auscultation médiate*.

Auscultation, though in practice and in our minds dating from Laennec and the invention of the stethoscope, was not an absolutely new idea in 1819. The Hippocratic School applied the ear to the chest and were familiar with pleuritic friction and succussion. Harvey listened to the sounds of the heart, Robert Boyle (1627–91) is said also to have done so, and a little later Robert Hooke (1605–1703), as told in his posthumous works published in 1705 by Richard Waller, listened to the heart and realized, but did not pursue, the possibilities of this method of obtaining information about the movements of the viscera. Laennec believed that G. L. Bayle (1774–1816), Corvisart's assistant when he worked under him, was the first of the moderns to practise the immediate or Hippocratic auscultation by putting his ear on the chest, and stated that Corvisart listened to the heart sounds with his ear very close to but not actually in contact with the chest wall. Double in 1817 advocated its adoption.

The story of the invention of the stethoscope by René Théophile Hyacinthe Laennec (1781–1826) has often been told: in 1816 he noticed boys in a Court of the Louvre at play with the ear applied to long pieces of wood listening to the transmitted sound of a pin scratch at the opposite end. He immediately put this hint into practice, as he says, by applying a rolled up quire of paper to the chest of a stout girl with symptoms of heart disease, and was electrified by finding that the heart sounds were more audible than to the direct ear. He keenly practised this method at the Necker Hospital, where, however, Granville, as an onlooker on 16 September 1816, states that the original birth of mediate auscultation actually occurred on the chest of a male patient. Laennec then devised a wooden cylinder $1\frac{1}{2}$ inches in diameter, a foot long, and perforated longitudinally by a bore three lines wide; this he regarded as too simple to require a name other than "the cylinder" or "bâton"; but eventually, as somewhat barbarous names, such as sonometra, pectorilogue, thoraciscope, cornet de papier, and cornet médical, appeared on the horizon, he suggested, if it must have a name, stethoscope. He gave an account of his

new method before the Académie des Sciences on
28 February 1818, and in May of the same year
lectured before the Medical Faculty of Paris. With
his knowledge of morbid anatomy he correlated the
local lesions with the corresponding physical signs,
like his teacher Corvisart, thus advancing the
anatomico-clinical method and the special pathology
of the organs, in the extraordinary short time of
three years, so that his classical work *Auscultation
médiate* appeared about 15 August 1819. While
correcting the proofs he had been busily making
stethoscopes so that every buyer of his book might
be properly equipped; in fact it is probable that at
the time of his death every existing stethoscope was
the work of his hand (Thayer).

Though the stethoscope has some obvious advantages over the naked ear, the enormous advances
that followed its introduction were not so much due
to the stethoscope as a mechanical instrument as to
the psychological effect that this new method exerted
on Laennec, who otherwise would not have so
ardently pursued auscultation as a means of diagnosis. It was much the same with regard to the
pleximeter introduced by P. A. Piorry (1794–1879)
(*Traité de la percussion médiate* dedicated "Aux
mânes d'Auenbrugger, de Corvisart, et de Laennec")
in 1828, which in itself, apart from its temporary
influence in stimulating investigation, is inferior as

a method of elicitating physical signs to Auenbrugger's direct percussion which it was intended to supersede; in 1866 Piorry, who was also a writer of verse, brought out his *Traité de plessimétriome et d'organographisme*, a volume of 750 pages.

Auscultation and percussion made their way somewhat slowly, and, as in the case of Harvey's discovery of the circulation, their appeal was to the young minds, such as John Forbes (1787–1861), James Jackson who in 1821 introduced it into the Massachusetts General Hospital, Boston, U.S.A. (Pratt), Thomas Hodgkin who in 1822 did the same at Guy's Hospital, Charles Scudamore (1779–1849) in *Observations on M. Laennec's Method*, etc. (1826), William Stokes (1804–78) of Dublin in his *Introduction to the Stethoscope* (1825), John Elliotson (1791–1868) in his *Lumleian Lectures*, 1829, on "Recent Improvements in the Art of Distinguishing the Various Diseases of the Heart", James Hope (1801–41), *A Treatise on Diseases of the Heart*, 1832, C. J. B. Williams (1805–89), a pupil of Laennec, who in 1828 dedicated his *Rational Exposition of the Physical Signs of Diseases of the Lungs and Pleura* to Sir Henry Halford, the President of the College, who, however, was never converted to the use of the stethoscope, and Thomas Davies (1792–1839) in his *Lectures on Diseases of the Heart and Lungs* (1835). It is rather remarkable that Sir Thomas

Watson (1792–1882) in his classical lectures (ed. 5
1871, vol. II, p. 20) says that the use of the stethoscope for auscultation is, with certain exceptions,
such as a dirty or infectious patient, "rather a
hindrance than a help". Laennec was more interested in the light thrown on pulmonary than on
cardiac disease, and the observations of some of the
authors just mentioned served to supplement and
extend his conclusions in this respect. Stimulated
by the appearance of Laennec's classic de Ker-
garadec in 1822 listened to the foetal heart; Mayor
of Geneva, however, had previously done this in
November 1818 (*vide* Forbes' translation of Laennec's *Auscultation médiate*, 1832, p. 714). But
deductions from auscultation of the heart were at
first under the grave disadvantage that the causes of
the first and second sounds were not correctly
known. Laennec attributed the first sound to the
contraction of the ventricles and the second to the
auricular systole; Laennec's error in the timing of
the second sound was pointed out by J. W. Turner
in 1828, and Hope, as the result of vivisection experiments performed at St George's Hospital
between 1830 and 1835, which gained for him the
distinction of the F.R.S. and an unfortunate con-
troversy as to priority with C. J. B. Williams,
eventually concluded that the first sound was due to
the muscular bruit and the tension of the auriculo-
ventricular valves and that the second sound was

due to the closure of the sigmoid valves. In 1836 and the following year a London Committee (C. J. B. Williams, R. B. Todd, and J. Clendinning) of the British Association for the Advancement of Science brought out reports "on the motions and sounds of the heart".[1]

Laennec's original stethoscope underwent modifications by him, Piorry who reduced the thickness of the stem to that of the finger, C. J. B. Williams, and others. The invention of the binaural was the subject of some dispute as to priority, as is shown in the pages of the *London Medical Gazette* for 1840–41; Sibson used one in 1838, Burne in 1840, and Golding Bird stated that Babington at Guy's had used one for some time. In America, where it was introduced in 1850 by Cammann, its vogue became general much earlier than in this country. Auscultatory percussion, or a combination of the two methods enabling

[1] In connection with the history of the heart sounds reference may be made to "the third sound" of the heart described by Einthoven, A. G. Gibson, and by Thayer (1909) in more than fifty per cent. of normal persons, especially under forty years of age, when lying on the left side. It occurs after the second sound in the early part of diastole, and has been ascribed to vibrations in the aortic valve segments (Einthoven) or to sudden tension in the auriculo-ventricular valves due to the rapid entry of blood into the ventricles (Thayer; A. G. Gibson). In certain circumstances the contraction of the auricle may give rise to a sound in diastole (G. A. Gibson and Malet).

the vibrations produced by percussion to be directly transmitted to the ear by the stethoscope, was advocated by Cammann and Clark in 1840. More modern developments are the phonendoscope and differential stethoscope.

Until auscultation had become somewhat elaborated the diagnosis of heart disease depended on general symptoms, such as dyspnoea, palpitation, a weak and irregular pulse, and there was not any discrimination in diagnosis. In the posthumous edition of Matthew Baillie's *Morbid Anatomy* (1825) it is stated that "no observations have yet been made by which practitioners can ascertain with any precision what set of valves is diseased". But Laennec's *Auscultation médiate* (1819) stirred the waters to much purpose. Bouillaud, Hope, Williams, and Elliotson became extremely active in tabulating the physical signs with the valvular lesions and accumulating data—the time, propagation, and characters—so as to determine the significance of murmurs. Hope's *A Treatise on Diseases of the Heart and Great Vessels*, 1832 (ed. 3, 1839), though somewhat marred by his disputes with Bouillaud, chronicled a most notable advance; having carried on experimental research, he was able to apply physiological principles to unravelling the haemo-dynamic problems of cardiac disease.

During the latter half of the last century an

exaggerated importance was attached to cardiac, and expecially systolic, murmurs as evidence of heart disease. With "the passing of morbid anatomy", or the overshadowing of gross morbid changes by the renewed attention to symptoms and physiological efficiency, there has now resulted a diminution in the importance attached to the physical signs of cardiac disease. But the traditional stress laid on the presence or absence of a murmur as the criteria in determining whether the heart was or was not affected, though qualified by the wise warnings of W. T. Gairdner (1862), Thomas Watson, Andrew Clark, G. W. Balfour, and others, did not become fully discounted until after the War, and then largely by Mackenzie's insistence. Indeed in 1914 medical officers recommended that soldiers with a systolic murmur should be discharged from the service. The great stress laid on diagnosis obscured the importance of prognosis, for which knowledge of the condition of efficiency of the myocardium is essential; but with the swing of the pendulum the myocardial factor is now well recognized in the principle that the diagnosis of valvular disease is determined by the auscultatory detection of murmurs, whereas its prognosis depends on the estimation of the myocardial efficiency.

The pulse rate. Although the ancient Egyptians, according to the Ebers papyrus (1600 B.C.), paid

R 6

attention to the pulse, and the Chinese in the fifth century B.C. attached great importance to the characters of the pulse, of which they recognized three thousand varieties, and Herophilus (300 B.C.) of Alexandria counted the pulse with his water clock or clepsydra, its rate apart from its other characters did not attract any general interest in Europe until long after Harvey's time. It is true that Sanctorius (1561–1636) in 1625 adapted Galileo's pulsometer (1582) to biological uses, but Harvey only refers to the pulse rate in the statement that it is from 1000 to 4000 in half an hour, and his junior contemporary Thomas Sydenham (1625–61) does not mention it. Sir John Floyer (1649–1734) in the *Physician's Pulse Watch*, or *An Essay to explain the old Art of feeling the Pulse*, in two volumes, the first of which appeared in 1707, the second in 1710, correctly predicted that his method of counting the pulse by a watch, which he constructed and set for sixty seconds, would be sneered at; indeed in 1772, eleven years after Morgagni reported a pulse of twenty-two in "the sixtieth of an hour", Théophile de Bordeu (1722–76), a fanciful theorist on endocrinology who elaborated many different pulses in the body, spoke of it somewhat contemptuously, and Falconer in 1798 remarked that "Floyer's methods were unused until now". In the meanwhile, however, there had been, not only in France but in Britain, much elaboration of unsupported detail current about the pulse and its significance, for example, R. Brookes in 1765 wrote "an intermitting pulse is, for the most part, full of danger and often fatal". This may have prompted William Heberden the elder to throw out a judicious warning and in 1768 to deprecate "minute distinctions in the pulse which chiefly exist in the imagination of the describers", and to state that an intermitting pulse is not dangerous, thus expressing the present view of extra-systoles. Corvisart in 1808 said little about the pulse rate. Caleb Hillier Parry's book in 1816, *An Experimental Inquiry into the Nature, Causes, and Varieties of the Arterial Pulse and into certain other Properties of the larger Arteries in Animals with warm Blood*, was an original and notable contribution. Hope in 1831 described the characters of the pulse in the various forms of valvular disease based on the examination of 10,000 patients between 1823 and 1829.

CARDIAC DYSPNOEA

As a result of work done during and since the War, cardiac dyspnoea may be divided into (i) simple, in which there is increased irritability of the respiratory centre from oxygen want brought about by diminished blood supply to the centre; in these cases, occurring in the young, especially with mitral stenosis, and comparatively early, the cyanosis being bright, Fraser, Ross and Dreyer found a definite alkalaemia, and Lewis and Barcroft noted the absence of acidaemia; (ii) cases of a more complicated nature, often arteriosclerotic or cardio-renal, in older people, with myocardial degeneration, dyspnoea occurring later and the cyanosis being of a leaden hue (Fraser). In these cases there is acidaemia (Lewis and Barcroft) and stimulation of the respiratory centre by the increased hydrogen-ion concentration, the fundamental idea that acidaemia causes breathlessness being directly deducible from Haldane and Priestley's work (1905). These cases manifest true cardiac asthma with a sudden onset which was ascribed by Lewis, Ryffel, Wolf, Cotton, and Barcroft (1913–14) to sudden waves of acidaemia. The attacks are probably much allied to those long known as renal asthma which, as pointed out by Loomis (1873) and Stephen Mackenzie (1889), are greatly benefited by hypodermic injection of morphine. These paroxysmal attacks of cardiac asthma were mentioned by Heberden, who eliminated from his picture of angina pectoris the symptoms of breathlessness; but there is a close relation between the three conditions of angina pectoris, oedema of the lung, and cardiac asthma (Pratt), which may be combined or confused with each other; in this connection it is interesting to note that Thomas Fowler

(1736–1801), whose name is so familiar in the solution of arsenic, wrote to William Withering a letter about his self-diagnosed angina pectoris, which Withering endorsed as asthma. Hope in his *Treatise* (1839) gave an account of cardiac asthma, but rather confused the issue by bringing in ordinary cardiac dyspnoea and Cheyne-Stokes respiration. Clinically James Mackenzie drew special attention to the true cardiac asthma about which scepticism had been expressed. The value of morphine hypodermically in the paroxysmal dyspnoea of cardiac asthma has recently been emphasized (Fraser), and it may be noted that on more general grounds Clifford Allbutt in 1869 recommended morphine in cardiac disease by the then comparatively new method of hypodermic injection, the syringe having been invented by Alexander Wood in 1855.

ANGINA PECTORIS

Angina pectoris[1] was first described on a good basis of cases, twenty in number, by the British Celsus,

[1] The correct pronunciation of the *i* in angina is short and not long as in general usage; this is settled, as scholars have been pointing out for some years, by the scansion in Plautus, *Trinummus*, II, iv, 139, Lucilius *ap.* Non. 35, 10, and Q. Serenus Samonicus, *de Medicina Praecepta*, v, 282 (*vide Brit. Med. Journ.* 1926, i, 1012, 1102). In an interesting note about this word, which is so much more familiar in modern medical than in

William Heberden the elder (1710–1801), in a paper entitled "Some Account of a Disorder of the Breast" read before this College on 21 July 1768, but not published until four years later. In the text he says: "The seat of it, and sense of strangling and anxiety with which it is attended, may make it not improperly called angina pectoris",[1] and his posthumous *Commentarii de Morborum Historia et Curatione*, 1802, p. 308, show that altogether he had seen a hundred cases. Isolated cases had been reported before this: Seneca in his epistles to Lucilius recorded his own sufferings, which may well have been those of angina sine dolore, and at any rate were by his medical attendants called a "Meditatio mortis", the Earl of Clarendon described the sudden death of his father Henry Hyde in 1632, and Morgagni the case of a woman who died in 1707 with a characteristic distribution of the pain and was found to have a dilated and calcified aorta. Hoffmann re-

classical works, J. W. Ogle (*St George's Hosp. Gaz.* 1899, VII, 141) quotes the evidence of the late Archbishop E. W. Benson to show that H. A. J. Munro, Professor of Latin in the University of Cambridge, made the discovery of the short *i* in angina early in 1879.

[1] In the 1780 edition of his *Primitive Physic, or an easy and Natural Method of curing most Diseases*, a popular hand-book written for the guidance of the poor, John Wesley translated angina pectoris into "quinsey of the breast".

corded another single case "de spasmo praecordiali
a motu corporis" in 1734; Rougnon, Professor of
Medicine in the University of Besançon, wrote a
letter to M. Lorry dated 23 February 1768, a copy
of which is in the library of the Surgeon-General of
the U.S. Army (Osler), earlier in the same year as
Heberden's more complete account, describing a
case of angina with a necropsy, and accordingly in
France a claim for priority was made for him by
Huchard. On 17 November 1772 two further communications on the subject were made to the
College; Heberden read a letter addressed to him by
a man signing himself "Unknown", who, having
seen an abstract of Heberden's original paper in
The Critical Review, recognized the resemblance to
his own experiences, gave an account of them, considered by Osler as one of the best extant, and
expressed a wish that in the event of his death there
should be a necropsy; this, when performed by John
Hunter, did not reveal anything save slight calcification of the aorta, but Edward Jenner, who was
present, wrote to Caleb Hillier Parry, "I can almost
positively say the coronary arteries of the heart were
not examined". The other, though less dramatic,
communication made at this meeting, by John Wall
(1708–76) of Worcester, has perhaps hardly received its due mead of attention; for in his letter to
Heberden describing the post-mortem examination

of a case of aortic stenosis with angina, the first inch of the aorta is stated to have been partly ossified, and the spasm of the pectoral muscle is ascribed to "an irritation on the nerves of the thorax and heart", and the following comment is added: "Perhaps it may throw some light on this affair to consider that the nervi intercostales or sympathetici distribute many branches to the heart, arteria pulmonalis, and aorta". He thus perhaps in the first place anticipated James Mackenzie's view that the pain of angina is partly due to spasm of the intercostal muscles and Charlton Briscoe's suggestion that the spread of pain depends upon irritation of one of the expiratory muscles, and in the second place suggested Corrigan's and Clifford Allbutt's conception of the aortic origin of anginoid pain. The association of coronary disease with angina was first recognized by Edward Jenner from post-mortem examination, though it is possible that John Hunter, on whose account, as his anginal symptoms dated from 1773, Jenner kept silence, knew or suspected it in 1776 when John Fothergill published a fatal case of angina in which at the post-mortem Hunter found that "the two coronary arteries from origin to many of their ramifications on the heart were become one piece of bone". Jenner, who is said to have diagnosed angina in Hunter in 1777 (*vide* Palmer), never directly published anything on this subject, but he communicated his opinions to C. H. Parry, who in 1788 read a paper, "An Inquiry into the Symptoms and Causes of the Syncope Anginosa, commonly called Angina Pectoris; illustrated by Dissections", to a small medical society in Gloucestershire of which Jenner was a member, and came to the conclusion that coronary disease was the cause. In this paper, not published until eleven years later, he quoted the case of ossification of the coronary arteries published by Black of Newry in 1795 and pointed out that he and Jenner had independently come to the same opinion in 1788.

The explanation of the causation of angina pectoris by coronary disease was, as pointed out by Osler, given by Allan Burns (1781–1813), the Glasgow anatomist and surgeon, who in 1809 ascribed the symptoms to anaemia, or as it might now be expressed anoxaemia, of the heart muscle resulting from coronary obstruction. This conception is now known as intermittent claudication—a term introduced by Bouley in 1831 in regard to horses and applied to man by Charcot in 1858—and perhaps more intelligibly as intermittent limp (Erb). Benjamin Brodie in 1846 explained angina pectoris on these lines rather more fully, and Potain in 1870 expressed the same opinion. The view that disease of the base of the aorta was one of the causes of angina pectoris, perhaps dimly foreshadowed by

Wall (1772) and Baumes of Montpellier (1808), was put forward by Dominic Corrigan (1802–80) in 1837, and by Clifford Allbutt from 1894, with confirmation from our Honorary Fellow, K. F. Wenckebach, in the special lecture he gave in this library on 5 May 1924, when he accordingly advocated division of the depressor nerve. James Mackenzie considered that angina is due to cardiac failure, a revival of the view held by Parry (1799) and supported by Stokes (1854), and Daniélopolu put forward the slightly different explanation that myocardial intoxication by fatigue products is responsible for angina.

The syndrome of angina pectoris, ascribed to various factors, has been divided into (i) true organic or major, and (ii) functional, pseudo, mock, false, vasomotorial or minor. John Latham (1812) described a spurious form as angina notha; Laennec, who had two attacks, did not accept coronary disease as the cause, considered mild cases as common, and described it as neuralgia of the heart; Desportes (1811) had previously expressed a similar view; Forbes, the translator of Laennec's *Auscultation médiate*, spoke of organic and of functional angina, subdividing these two main categories. Lartigue (1846) and Walshe independently introduced the term "pseudo-angina", which has not escaped criticism from Allbutt and Mackenzie; Nothnagel in 1867 brought in the term vasomotor angina; and toxic angina, especially that due to tobacco, was described by Huchard. Angina sine dolore, a form of true or major angina, was so named by W. T. Gairdner (1877). The distribution of pain and cutaneous tenderness was investigated by James Mackenzie (1892) and Henry Head.

Excision of the cervico-thoracic sympathetic containing the sensory nerves of the heart and aorta as a means of relieving the pain of angina was suggested in 1899 by François-Franck, the physiologist, but not put into practice until 1916 by Jonnesco of Bucarest. The treatment by amyl nitrite was initiated in 1867 by Lauder Brunton (1844–1916), when a house physician, on the grounds that he found the blood pressure high in an attack and, having heard from Arthur Gamgee that amyl nitrite lowered the blood pressure, logically and successfully employed this drug.

In the tercentenary year of the publication of the *De Motu Cordis* it is interesting to find that the coronary circulation, on which R. Lower, R. Vieussens (1706, 1715), and Adam Christian Thebesius (1708) worked, has been investigated after the Harveian manner. Wearn finds that the blood in the coronary arteries may pass into the Thebesian vessels and so into the ventricles or auricles without entering the capillaries, there being either a direct communication between the coronary arteries and the Thebesian veins, or more probably between the arteries and large veins, and thence into the cavities of the heart. Further, he argues from observations on two cases of gradual complete obliteration of the orifices of both coronary arteries that the Thebesian vessels may take on the new function of supplying the heart muscle with blood from the cavities of the heart, a view to some extent previously expressed by Pratt. The coronary blood flow depends on the arterial pressure, but opinions differ as to the relative importance of the diastolic and systolic blood pressures in the aorta. In this year Anrep and King have shown by experiment that the coronary blood flow is not determined by either the diastolic or the systolic pressures in the aorta singly, but follows closely changes in the arithmetical average of the diastolic and systolic aortic pressures, which in most cases is a sufficiently accurate measure of the true mean pressure.

CORONARY THROMBOSIS

The syndrome of thrombosis of the coronary arteries, long included in angina, has quite recently been isolated, though Harvey's description of Sir Robert Darcy's case, in his second Disquisition to J. Riolan, in which the wall of the left ventricle was ruptured apparently as the result of "an impediment to the passage of the blood from the left ventricle into the arteries", has now been recognized as an early example (Wearn). The syndrome, first described in 1910 by Obrastzow and Strachesko and again in 1912 by J. B. Herrick, is, now that its characteristic features have been pointed out, obviously a frequent event; this year Parkinson and Bedford published one hundred clinical cases and in addition eighty-three post-mortem cases. Isolated cases had been reported in 1884 by Leyden and even diagnosed by Hammer in 1878, and it is now easy to wonder why coronary occlusion, long recognized pathologically, had not been correlated earlier with a clinical picture. Cases of angina with pericarditis had been recorded (Steell), and the occurrence of the status anginosus, or pain lasting for hours or days in contrast to the pain of angina, which is a matter of minutes, was noted by Huchard. Both these phenomena belong to the syndrome of coronary thrombosis. Rapid and sudden death may be due to ventricular fibrillation or to rupture of the infarcted area as in Harvey's case; recovery may occur, but myocardial failure, cardiac aneurysm, rupture, or recurrent thrombosis may follow.

STOKES-ADAMS SYNDROME

J. B. Morgagni in 1761 mentioned two men aged sixty-eight and sixty-four years with slow pulse-rates, one "twenty-two within one-sixtieth part of

an hour", dating from the time they were "first
attacked with epileptic paroxysms, beginning from
the belly"; Heberden in 1768 described a pulse
seldom above thirty associated with torpidity;
Andrew Duncan described the same events in 1793;
Bright in 1831 recorded the clinical features of a case
with a necropsy showing a much enlarged heart.
The condition was called maladie de Stokes-Adams
by Huchard after the two Irish physicians, Robert
Adams and William Stokes, who gave accounts of it
in 1827 and 1846 respectively and laid much stress
on fatty degeneration of the myocardium; indeed,
they transferred to that condition many of the
symptoms of complete heart-block. This of course
was long before Gaskell's physiological explanation
(1883) of heart-block which is usually, but not invariably, primarily responsible for the syndrome.
Galabin in 1875 first published tracings of the independent contractions of the auricles and ventricles, and ten years later Chauveau's tracings also
showed this in a man with an auricular rate of sixty
to sixty-five and a ventricular rate of twenty-one to
twenty-four. Osler pointed out the various forms
of the Stokes-Adams syndrome, especially the rare
cases with gross extrinsic lesions exerting pressure
on the medulla or the vagus, such as those of
Holberton, Lépine, and Boffard, and to his writings
the general recognition of the syndrome is due in no

small degree. Recently it has been shown that the ventricle may pass into fibrillation, and that the direct injection of adrenaline into the heart will start the circulation again even if it has stopped for four or five minutes. Subcutaneous injection of adrenaline has been found to arrest the syncopal attacks (Phear and Parkinson) but not to prevent them. For this purpose Cohn and Levine had recourse to barium chloride by the mouth, which, by increasing the irritability of the ventricle, was successful in preventing the attacks. An interesting account of his own experiences during the last seven years of his life was given by W. T. Gairdner (1824–1907).

EXOPHTHALMIC GOITRE

Exophthalmic goitre, which had been erroneously regarded as aneurysm by Aetius (A.D. 500) and by Ambroise Paré (1561), was observed by Caleb Hillier Parry (1755–1822) of Bath first in 1786, but not published until 1825 under the title of *Enlargement of the Thyroid Gland in connection with Enlargement or Palpitation of the Heart*, when eight cases were retailed; he wrote, "my attendance on the three last patients having occurred at the same time (1813) first suggested to me the notion of some connection between the malady of the heart and the bronchocele". His full recognition of the disease thus came some twenty-seven years after he first saw a case.

Two of his case reports (Nos. 3 and 8), one of a patient "long affected with an extremely large swelling of the thyroid gland, which began at a period, the relation of which to the commencement of the disorder of the heart, she was unable to re-collect", and of the other who had "had an enlargement of the thyroid gland for more than twenty years which has very much increased of late", may have been what would now be called a toxic adenoma. Osler piously called the disease after "the distinguished old Bath physician". In Italy it has been called Flajani's disease after the describer in 1800, thus anticipating by many years R. J. Graves' description in 1835, and Karl A. von Basedow of Merseberg's account of the three most important symptoms ("the Merseberg triad") in 1840. This is the richest disease in eponyms, but three of the eight known, Parsons', Marsh's (Sir Henry Marsh (1790–1860) of Dublin), and Stokes' disease have long ceased to be employed.

REFERENCES

II

Percussion and Auscultation:

BAILLIE, M. Works Edited by James Wardrop. 1825. Vol. II.
—— The Morbid Anatomy of some of the most important Parts of the Human Body. P. 43.
BIRD, G. *London Med. Gaz.* 1840–41, N.S. II, 510.

BURNE, J. *Ibid.* 1840–41, N.S. II, 468.

CAMMANN and CLARK. *New York Journ. Med. and Surg.* 1840, III, 62.

DOUBLE, F. J. Seméiologie générale, ou traité des signes et de leur valeur dans les maladies. 1817. Tome II, p. 186.

EINTHOVEN, W. *Arch. f. d. ges. Physiol.* 1907, CXX, 31.

GAIRDNER, W. T. *Edin. Med. Journ.* 1861–2, VII, 438.

GIBSON, A. G. *Lancet*, London, 1907, ii, 1380.

GIBSON, G. A. and MALET. *Journ. Anat. and Physiol.* London, 1879, XIV, 1.

GRANVILLE, A. B. Sudden Death. 1854.

PRATT, J. H. *Boston Med. and Surg. Journ.* 1925, CXCIII, 200.

SIBSON, F. *London Med. Gaz.* 1840–41, N.S. II, 911.

THAYER, W. S. *Boston Med. and Surg. Journ.* 1908, CLVIII, 713; and *Arch. Int. Med.* 1909, IV, 297.

—— "Some Unpublished Letters of Laennec," *Bull. Johns Hopkins Hosp.* Baltimore, 1920, XXXI, 427.

TURNER, J. W. *Trans. Med.-Chir. Soc. Edin.* 1828, III, 205.

WILLIAMS, C. J. B. Rational Exposition of the Physical Signs of Diseases of the Lungs and Pleura. 1828.

The Pulse Rate:

BROOKES, R. The General Practice of Physic extracted chiefly from the writings of the most famous Physicians. 1765. Vol. I, p. 52.

DE BORDEU, T. Recherches sur le pouls par rapport aux crises. 1772.

HEBERDEN, W. *Med. Trans. Coll. Phys. Lond.* 1772, II, 18.

MORGAGNI, J. B. De Sedibus et Causis Morborum, 1761.

Cardiac Dyspnoea:

ALLBUTT, T. C. *Practitioner*, 1869, III, 342.

FRASER, F. R. *Lancet*, London, 1927, i, 429, 589, 643.

FRASER, ROSS and DREYER. *Quart. Journ. Med.* Oxford, 1821–2, XV, 195.

HALDANE and PRIESTLEY. *Journ. Physiol.* Cambridge, 1905, XXXII, 225.

HEBERDEN, W. Commentaries on the History and Cure of Disease. 1803. P. 68.

HOPE, J. A Treatise on Diseases of the Heart and Great Vessels. 1839. P. 395.

LEWIS and BARCROFT. *Quart. Journ. Med.* Oxford, 1914–15, VIII, 97.

98   UNAIDED CLINICAL OBSERVATION

LEWIS, RYFFEL, WOLF, COTTON and BARCROFT. *Heart*, London, 1913–14, v, 45.
LOOMIS, A. L. *Med. Rec.* N.Y. 1873, VIII, 364.
MACKENZIE, J. *Brit. Med. Journ.* 1911, ii, 1231.
MACKENZIE, S. *Lancet*, London, 1889, ii, 208.
PRATT, J. H. *Journ. Am. Med. Assoc.* Chicago, 1926, LXXXVII, 809.
WOOD, A. A New Method of Treating Neuralgia by Subcutaneous Injection. 1855.

Angina Pectoris:

ALLBUTT, T. C. Diseases of the Arteries including Angina Pectoris. 1915. Vol. II, 416.
ANREP, G. V. and KING, B. *Journ. Physiol.* Cambridge, 1928, LXIX, 341.
BAUMES. *Ann. Soc. de méd. prat. de Montpel.* 1808, XII, 225.
BLACK, S. *Mem. Med. Soc. London*, 1795, IV, 261.
BOULEY, H. (Jeune). *Arch. de méd.* Paris, 1831, s. 1, XXVII, 425.
BRISCOE, C. *Lancet*, London, 1921, ii, 1257.
BRODIE, B. Lectures illustrative of Pathology and Surgery. 1846. P. 361.
BRUNTON, T. L. *Lancet*, London, 1867, ii, 97.
BURNS, ALLAN. Observations on some of the Most Frequent and Important Diseases of the Heart. 1809. P. 136.
CHARCOT, J. M. *Compt. rend. Soc. biol.* 1858, Paris, 1859, s. 2, v, part 2, 225.
CLARENDON, EDWARD, Earl of. Life written by himself. Oxford, 1759. P. 9.
CORRIGAN, D. *Dublin Journ. Med. Sc.* 1837, XII, 243.
DANIÉLOPOLU, D. L'angine de poitrine. 1924.
ERB. *Deutsche Ztschr. f. Nervenh.* Leipzig, 1898, XIII, 1.
FORBES, J. Cyclopaedia Pract. Med. 1833. Vol. I, p. 87.
FOTHERGILL, J. *Med. Observ. and Inquir.* 1776, v, 152.
GAIRDNER, W. T. System of Medicine (Russell Reynolds). 1877. Vol. IV, p. 554.
HEAD, H. *Brain*, London, 1893, XVI, 56.
HEBERDEN, W. *Med. Trans. Coll. Phys. Lond.* 1772, II, 59.
—— *Ibid.* 1785, III, 1–11.
HOFFMANN, F. Consultationum et Responsorum medicinalium Centuria prima, complectens Morbos Capitis et Pectoris. Vol. I. 1734.
HUCHARD, H. Traité des maladies du cœur, etc. 1889.

LARTIGUE, A. Mémoire sur l'angine de la poitrine. Paris, 1846.

LATHAM, J. *Med. Trans. Coll. Phys. Lond.* 1813, IV, 278.

MACKENZIE, J. *Med. Chron.* Manchester, 1892, XVI, 293.

—— Angina Pectoris. London, 1923.

MORGAGNI. De Sedibus et Causis Morborum. 1762. Lib. II, Epist. XXI, 31.

NOTHNAGEL, H. *Deutsches Arch. f. klin. Med.* 1867, III, 309.

OSLER, W. Lectures on Angina Pectoris and Allied States. 1897. P. 7.

PALMER, J. F. The Works of John Hunter, with Notes. 1837. Vol. I, p. 64.

PARRY, C. H. An Inquiry into the Symptoms and Causes of the Syncope Anginosa, etc. London, 1799. 8vo.

PRATT, F. H. *Am. Journ. Physiol.* 1898, I, 86.

THEBESIUS, A. C. Dissertatio medica de circulo sanguinis in corde. Lugduni Batavorum, 1708.

VIEUSSENS, R. Nouvelles découvertes sur le cœur. Toulouse, 1706.

—— Traité nouveau de la substance et des causes des mouvements du cœur. Toulouse, 1715.

WALL, J. *Med. Trans. Coll. Phys. Lond.* 1785, III, 12.

WALSHE, W. H. Diseases of the Heart and Great Vessels, 1862.

WEARN, J. T. *Journ. Exper. Med.* 1928, XLVII, 293.

WENCKEBACH, K. F. *Brit. Med. Journ.* 1924, i, 809.

Coronary Thrombosis:

HAMMAN, L. *Bull. Johns Hopkins Hosp.*, Baltimore, 1926, XXXVIII, 273 (literature).

HARVEY, W. Works of, Translated by R. Willis, Sydenham Society. 1847. P. 127.

HERRICK, J. B. *Journ. Am. Med. Assoc.* Chicago, 1912, LIX, 2015.

HUCHARD, H. Traité des maladies du cœur et des vaisseaux. Paris, 1899. Vol. II, p. 128.

McNEE, J. W. *Quart. Journ. Med.* Oxford, 1925–6, XIX, 44.

OBRASTZOW, W. P. und STRACHESKO, N. D. *Ztschr. f. klin. Med.* 1910, LXXI, 116.

PARKINSON and BEDFORD. *Lancet*, London, 1928, i, 4 (and history).

STEELL, G. *Med. Chron.* Manchester, 1913–14, LVIII, 97.

WEARN, J. T. *Am. Journ. Med. Sc.* Phila. 1923, CLXV, 250.

Stokes-Adams Syndrome:

ADAMS, R. *Dublin Hosp. Rep.* 1827, IV, 396.

BRIGHT, R. Reports of Medical Cases. 1831. Vol. II, part i, p. 270.

CHAUVEAU, A. *Rev. de méd.* Paris, 1885, v, 161.

COHN and LEVINE. *Arch. Int. Med.* Chicago, 1925, XXXVI, 1.

DUNCAN, A. *Vide* W. T. Ritchie, *Edin. Med. Journ.* 1923, N.S. XXX, 621.

GAIRDNER, W. T. Life of, pp. 138–152, by G. A. Gibson. 1912.

GALABIN, A. L. *Guy's Hosp. Rep.* 1875, s. 3, XX, 280.

HEBERDEN, W. *Med. Trans. Coll. Phys. Lond.* 1772, II, 30.

HUCHARD, H. Traité des maladies du cœur et des vaisseaux. Paris, 1889. P. 255.

LEVINE and MATTON. *Heart*, 1926, XII, 271.

MORGAGNI, J. B. De Sedibus et Causis Morborum. 1761. Book II, Letter 24, Art. 33.

OSLER, W. Lectures on Angina and Allied States. 1897. P. 70.

—— *Lancet*, London, 1903, ii, 516.

PHEAR and PARKINSON. *Ibid.* 1922, i, 933.

STOKES, W. *Dublin Quart. Journ. Med. Sc.* 1846, ii, 73–85.

III

Examination of Patients with the Aid of Instruments of Precision

UNDER this heading brief reference will be made to the history of sphygmomano-meters, sphygmographs, X-ray assistance, the electrocardiograph, and to some cardiac disorders the nature of which has been determined by in-strumental assistance. In addition, a short note on the early history of digitalis is appended.

Sphygmomanometry. The history of blood pressure really begins with Stephen Hales (1677–1761), minister of Teddington, who with a sound training in Newtonian physics applied this knowledge to biology and physiology. Before 1723 he tied tubes into the arteries and veins of animals and estimated the pressure in the capillaries, thus being far in advance of his time. In a mare he found that the blood pressure was equal to a column of blood of eight to nine feet. Nearly a century passed before the subject was further investigated, and then Poiseuille (1828) employed a **U**-shaped mercurial manometer (haemodynometer) which, as van Leer-sum points out, was but a step from the mercurial column used by Hales to estimate the pressure of the sap in a pruned vine. To this, in 1847, Carl Ludwig added a float with a pen to record the variations of the blood pressure on a revolving cylinder (kymograph). Experimental methods of estimating the arterial blood pressure then were pursued by a number of observers, such as A. Fick (1864, 1885) with a spring manometer, Marey's sphygmoscope (1875) modified by Hürthle into a rubber manometer, and von Frey's metal tonograph.

In the meanwhile Bright (1836) had noticed the hard pulse in renal disease as judged by the finger, and he has been called "the first student of the hypertensive problem" (Janeway). The clinical estimation of blood pressure by instrumental means was first attempted by Vierordt in 1855 by measuring the weight necessary to stop the arterial pulsation; but von Basch in 1880 invented a sphygmomanometer on this principle which was applied locally over an artery and was widely used. This underwent modifications, among others by Potain (1889); Marey compressed the whole of the forearm, later confining this method to the finger; Mosso and Hürthle also introduced modifications. Attention should be drawn to F. A. Mahomed's laborious observations on blood pressure made between 1874 and 1881, not with a sphygmomanometer but with his own form of Marey's sphygmograph, which led him to anticipate much that is now known and far more easily verified; for example, he described a pre-albuminuric rise of blood pressure in Bright's disease, which with von Basch's conception of "latent arteriosclerosis" and Huchard's pre-sclerosis led up to the recognition of primary or essential high blood pressure or hyperpiesia. The present sphygmomanometric methods became generally available as a result of Riva-Rocci's modification of von Basch's instrument with a piece of rubber tubing to surround the arm in 1897, and by Hill and Barnard's independent description of a somewhat similar instrument in the same year. Gaertner's tonometer took the pressure by means of an elastic bag enclosing the finger (1889). In 1901 von Recklinghausen showed that as a result of the insufficient width of the rubber tube armlets a higher systolic pressure was registered than actually existed; this was confirmed by C. J. Martin and remedied in his mercurial sphygmomanometer (1905), Mummery's, and other modifications of the Riva-Rocci model. Numerous other forms of pressure gauges were introduced by G. A. Gibson, Erlanger, Cook, Stanton, and Pachon. The publication of Korotkoff's auditory or auscultatory method in 1905 has made estimation of the diastolic pressure both easy and accurate for all conditions except some cases of aortic regurgitation.

The general use of the sphygmomanometer in this country was largely due to Clifford Allbutt,

Brunton, and G. Oliver. The greater stability of the diastolic than of the systolic pressure, and therefore its greater diagnostic value, the importance of the pulse or differential pressure, and a correct estimation of the significance of abnormal pressures have gradually become stablished. Clifford Allbutt described the occurrence of high blood pressure without renal disease, and introduced for this the word hyperpiesia. He also insisted that long-continued high blood pressure may cause, but is not due to, arteriosclerosis.

Estimation of the venous pressure and of the capillary blood pressure has naturally followed; Hooker's water manometer applied to the veins of the hand shows that normally it is not above 10 mm. of water, and that in cardiac failure it is raised to twice or thrice this figure. A rise or fall in the venous pressure may indicate improvement or a relapse in the cardiac condition before this is clinically evident (A. H. Clark). Venesection naturally lowers the venous pressure, but a rapid rise after bleeding is said to point to a low reserve power in the heart (Eyster and Middleton). The capillary blood pressure can be measured by Danzer and Hooker's microcapillary tonometer and shown to be normally 100–200 mm. H_2O. It is not raised in hyperpiesia (without renal disease) or in chronic interstitial nephritis, but is raised in glomerulo-nephritis (Kylin).

The sphygmograph, first invented by K. Vierordt in 1855, and improved by Marie (1860), who did so much to popularize the method of graphic registration, Mahomed (1872), Burdon-Sanderson (1867), R. E. Dudgeon (1882), Pond, von Jacquet, and others, was much used; though the information it provided was somewhat limited, it was the first step in the application to cardiology of the graphic method of record, which has since thrown so much light on haemo-dynamics. By means of his clinical polygraph James Mackenzie (1902), then of Burnley, correlated the arterial and venous pulses with those of the heart, and thus brought order out of the chaos of cardiac irregularities, distinguishing the unimportant, such as the extra-systoles of sinus arrhythmia, from those, such as pulsus alternans, pathognomonic of grave organic disease of the heart muscle. Thus he recognized the completely irregular heart, which was later shown to be due to fibrillation of the auricles. This last advance came from the application to medicine of another physiological instrument, the string galvanometer, aided by animal experiment. As a method of investigation the sphygmograph has been largely superseded by the string galvanometer, except as regards the detection of the pulsus alternans.

The advent of *radiology* enabled the size, shape, and condition of the heart to be much more accurately determined than by percussion, and the employment of the fluorescent screen (orthodiagraphy), X-ray films taken in the ordinary way or at preferably a distance of two metres (teleoroentgenogram) to avoid error of distortion, has been of such enormous assistance in clinical diagnosis, especially as regards that of a deep-seated aneurysm, that there is a risk that ordinary percussion will be neglected.

The electrocardiograph. The potential bearings of investigating the electric currents produced by the cardiac contractions, recognized in 1843 by Matteuci of Pisa and in 1856 by Kölliker and Müller, were examined with the capillary electrometer by Sanderson and Page (1878), Gaskell (1881), Starling and Bayliss (1890), and A. D. Waller. In 1903 Willem Einthoven (1860–1927) of Leyden first described the string galvanometer which was a great advance on the capillary and other galvanometers, and utilizing Waller's observation that curves of the cardiac contractions can be obtained from the limbs of animals without opening the chest, he, as Sir Thomas Lewis says, laid the foundation of human and experimental electrocardiography and by papers published in 1907 and 1908 led to modern electrocardiography and the final analysis of the arrhythmias. The fundamental knowledge thus acquired by methods demanding delicate instruments it has fortunately been possible to correlate in many instances with simple indications which can be employed at the bedside. Wenckebach, Thomas Lewis, and their followers have thus exactly localized the site of disorders and morbid changes in different parts of the heart muscle, and particularly in the junctional system, such as lesions of the right or left branch of the auriculo-ventricular bundle, and the Purkinje arborizations, thus providing evidence of myocardial degeneration and impending cardiac failure earlier than can be detected by other means of examination (*vide* Oppenheimer and Rothschild).

Auricular flutter was described as long ago as 1887 by MacWilliam as the result of weak faradization of the mammalian auricles. Clinically, however, it was not recognized until much later by W. T. Ritchie and by Hertz and Goodhart. A healthy auricle responds to a single stimulus by a single contraction; but if the refractory period of a ring of muscle, as in the auricles, is shortened, the wave of contraction travels round continuously and is spoken of as a circus movement. This physiological observation of G. R. Mines was further elucidated as the condition in auricular flutter by Thomas Lewis and his co-workers. The auricles contract extremely rapidly —200 to 300 or more times a minute, the ventricular rate being usually half that. The treatment consists in the production of a certain degree of heart block by digitalis, or more radically by directly acting on the muscular tissue of the auricle by quinidine sulphate.

The development of knowledge about *auricular fibrillation*[1] illustrates the close interdependence of clinical medicine and experimental work. Auricular fibrillation, long familiar to physiologists was first recognized in man by Cushny and Edmunds in a case under their care in 1901 and published in 1906, the fibrillation being ascribed to vagal inhibition; but their diagnosis of fibrillation was received with doubt. In 1902 Mackenzie had recognized the complete irregularity of the pulse now known to be characteristic of auricular fibrillation, and on the ground of the absence of the auricular wave in the jugular tracings argued that the auricles had ceased to contract and were paralysed. In 1907 he abandoned the idea of paralysis, as in some cases at any rate the muscular fibres of the auricles were found by Keith to be hypertrophied, and argued that the auricular and ventricular contractions occurred simultaneously as the result of irritability of the auriculo-ventricular node, and called this "nodal rhythm". In 1910 Rothberger and Winterberg, and Lewis, by means of the electrocardiograph, proved

[1] Historically it is of interest that retrospective diagnosis has led H. B. Anderson to ascribe the death of the poet Robert Burns, not to alcoholism, but to rheumatic heart disease, auricular fibrillation, and terminal bacterial endocarditis, the last two being, according to Rothschild, Sacks, and Libman, so rarely combined as to be mutually exclusive.

that the auricular condition was one of auricular fibrillation. The condition of nodal rhythm or simultaneous contractions of the auricles and ventricles due to the stimulus starting in the auricular ventricular instead of in the sino-auricular node occurs but is uncommon.

Auricular flutter and auricular fibrillation are closely related and in the same heart one may be transformed into the other; thus under quinidine fibrillation returns through impure and occasionally pure flutter to a normal rhythm (Lewis, Drury, Iliescu and Wedd). They are both due to circus movement in the auricles depending on shortening of the refractory period in the muscle fibres. But in auricular fibrillation the refractory period of the muscle is shorter and as a result the path taken by the circus movement is therefore shorter and more irregular than in flutter (Lewis, 1921). The muscle fibres of the auricle contract independently of each other and much more rapidly than in flutter. The auricle fibrillating at the rate of 450 times a minute overwhelms the conducting capacity of the auriculo-ventricular bundle, so that some only of the impulses reach the ventricle, and these are so irregular that the characteristic pulse results.

Quinidine sulphate and digitalis relieve the subjects of auricular fibrillation in different ways; Mackenzie showed the value of digitalis in auricular fibrillation while recognizing that it did not restore the auricular contractions, and Cushny and others proved that it acted by inducing a certain amount of heart block. An enormous amount of experimental work has been done upon the action of digitalis on the heart of cold and warm blooded animals, the effects on the two being different. In the mammalian heart contractility and inhibition are increased and then conduction is impaired. The slowing of the pulse is mainly due, as Traube showed in 1851 by section of the vagi, to stimulation of the inhibitory centre in the medulla, and is abolished by the action of atropine (Ackermann). Dixon's experiments suggest that this vagal stimulation leads to the production in the nerve ending of a substance resembling muscarine, which by combining with a body in the myocardium brings about inhibition. Eggleston's rapid method of giving the necessary amount of digitalis, as estimated by the body weight, in three doses at six-hour intervals has given good results in suitable cases (Fraser).

Quinine was found by Wenckebach in 1914 to restore the normal rhythm in auricular fibrillation, and W. von Frey, after trying the various cinchona derivatives, found that quinidine, which was first isolated by van Heijningen in 1849 and in 1853 by Pasteur, in perhaps a purer form, gave far the best results in flutter and auricular fibrillation. The ob-

servations of Lewis and his co-workers upon the
action of certain drugs upon fibrillation of the
auricles in 1922 showed that quinidine sulphate
lengthens the refractory period and so, by closing
the gap between the wake and the advance of the
circulating way, tends to abolish auricular fibrillation; but in addition it has the antagonistic effect of
slowing conduction and so widening the gap between
the successive waves. Successful treatment therefore depends on the first effect being predominant,
and so enabling the normal pace-maker to regain
control. While powerful for good, quinidine exerts
untoward effects by detaching clots and causing
embolism, and may poison the myocardium, causing
ventricular tachycardia passing into ventricular
fibrillation.

Ventricular fibrillation was described as a cause of
sudden death in man by MacWilliam in 1889,
following on Ludwig and Hoffa's demonstration in
1850 that the application of strong electric currents
to the ventricles of a frog's heart set up fibrillary
contractions, and Kronecker's production of a
similar condition by puncture of a point of the
interventricular septum.

Paroxysmal tachycardia was described by Cotton
(1867), called tachycardia by Gerhardt (1881), received its full title from Bouveret (1889), and was
critically considered by Herringham (1897). The

polygraph and the electrocardiograph in Mackenzie and Lewis' hands have thrown much light on this clinical syndrome, showing that it is not simply an acceleration of rate, but that the rhythm is abnormal as a result of the stimulus originating not in the sino-auricular node but elsewhere. The ectopic stimulus may start in the auricle, so that transient attacks may be due to accelerated nodal rhythm (Lewis), to auricular flutter, to auricular fibrillation, or may even originate in the ventricle.

THE HISTORY OF DIGITALIS

Unlike squills, familiar to the Hippocratic School, digitalis was unknown to the Greeks and Romans, and the earliest reference to it from a medical point of view is stated to be in a list of herbs for the Myddvai medical men of Wales in the thirteenth century (D. McKenzie). Leonard Fuchs of Tübingen described it in 1542 and named it digitalis either from its French name, *herbe à doigt*, or as a translation of *fingerhut* = thimble; its English name has been derived from Folk's (the fairies) glove (Balfour) or possibly from the describer's name (Fuchs = fox), as Vaquez suggests. It was mentioned by the herbalists John Gerard (1597) and John Parkinson (1640) for its expectorant, emetic, and anti-epileptic properties. After finding a place among the simples in the London pharmacopoeias of 1650, 1678, 1682, and 1721, it disappeared from that list in 1746, but was reinstated in 1788, and in 1809 was supplemented by an account of its tincture and infusion. Von Helmont, Boerhaave, and Haller applied it externally for scrofula; but generally speaking it was employed in the King's Evil and epilepsy rather because it was a herb of grace than for its clinical influence, and orthodox practitioners did not take its claims seriously. On the other hand, it was in vogue among wise women for dropsy, especially for that below the waist.

Professional attention to its remedial action of course was really due to the advocacy of William Withering[1] (1741–99), physician (1779–92) to the General Hospital, Birmingham, and closely associated with Thomas Fowler (1736–1801) of Stafford, whose name is perpetuated in connection with another drug of undoubted value, liquor arsenicalis. Settling in Birmingham in 1775, Withering took the house formerly occupied by Dr Robert

[1] The portrait of Withering painted by C. F. von Breda, painter to the King of Sweden, in 1792, when visiting Edgbaston, which was reproduced in *The Miscellaneous Tracts of the late William Withering, M.D., F.R.S.*, edited by his son William Withering, 2 vols. 1822, and by A. R. Cushny in *The Action and Uses in Medicine of Digitalis and its Allies*, 1925, and by W. H. Wynn in his memoir of Withering (*Birmingham Med. Rev.* 1926, N.S. 1), is now, Dr W. E. Dixon tells me, in the National Gallery at Stockholm.

James (1705–76), author of the *Medical Dictionary* (1743) in which Samuel Johnson wrote, and responsible for the famous fever powder. In 1775 Withering's opinion was sought about a secret remedy for dropsy composed of twenty or more herbs, of which he recognized that foxglove was the only one likely to be effective; he therefore tried it in practice, and it thus began to be used by his local colleagues; in 1779 Dr Stokes of Stourbridge brought its use by Withering before the Medical Society of Edinburgh, which led to its use in the Royal Infirmary and its inclusion in the *Edinburgh Pharmacopoeia* of 1783 before the appearance in 1785 of Withering's *Account of Foxglove and its Medicinal Uses with practical Remarks on Dropsy and other Diseases*. In the light of its use in Edinburgh it is rather remarkable that Samuel Johnson, when suffering from dropsy in 1784, obtained through Boswell the advice of five Edinburgh physicians— Sir Alexander Dick, Drs Gillespie, William Cullen, John Hope, and Alexander Monro *secundus*—he was not given digitalis, but rhubarb grown in the garden of the octogenarian Sir Alexander Dick. Erasmus Darwin in 1780, in an appendix to the thesis of his son Charles and again in 1785, wrote on its uses in dropsy.

Withering did not ascribe its diuretic effect to its action on the heart, though he noted that "it has a

power over the motion of the heart to a degree yet
unobserved in any other medicine, and that this
power may be converted to salutary ends", a
reduction of the pulse rate to thirty-five per minute.
William Cullen (1789) suggested that its diuretic
effect was connected with a general influence on the
body as manifested by the slowing of the pulse.
John Ferriar of Manchester in 1799 insisted on its
power of reducing the pulse, and recommended it in
cardiac palpitation, oedema of the lungs, general
dropsy, and haemoptysis. The administration of
digitalis gradually became the routine treatment of
heart disease, while its use in pulmonary tuberculosis
was abandoned. In 1845 Homolle and Quevenne
isolated digitaline. Attention should be recalled to
Lauder Brunton's M.D. thesis *On Digitalis with some
Observations on the Urine* (1866), based on six months'
observations on himself. There was really little
advance in the selection of cases for treatment during
the nineteenth century, and two clinical views—that
it raises the blood pressure and that it must never
be given in aortic regurgitation—arose during the
latter half of this period; indeed, as Cushny said,
it was not until the physiological work and con-
ceptions of Gaskell were applied to medicine by
James Mackenzie and K. F. Wenckebach that any
real advance was made on the knowledge of digitalis
and its uses a century earlier. A very important

step, from a practical point of view, was the demonstration by Sahli in 1901 that therapeutic doses do not raise the blood pressure in man, as had been generally assumed on the evidence of the experimental administration of massive doses to animals by James Blake (1839), Brunton and Meyer (1873), Donaldson and Stevens (1883), and others. The fear of giving digitalis in cardiac failure with high blood pressure and arteriosclerosis, and so further increasing the work of the heart and of causing cerebral haemorrhage, was not allayed in this country until much later, and then as the result of James Mackenzie's insistence. Standardization of digitalis preparations has been an important step towards effective treatment.

REFERENCES

III

Sphygmomanometers:

ALLBUTT, T. C. Diseases of Arteries including Angina Pectoris. 1915.
BRIGHT, R. *Guy's Hosp. Rep.* 1836, I, 338.
CLARK, A. H. *Arch. Int. Med.* Chicago, 1915, XVI, 587.
EYSTER, J. A. E. and MIDDLETON, W. S. *Am. Journ. Med. Sc.* Phila. 1927, CLXXIV, 486.
HALES, S. Haemastatics. 1733. Vol. II, p. 3.
HILL, L. and BARNARD, H. L. *Brit. Med. Journ.* 1897, ii, 904.
HOOKER, D. R. and EYSTER, J. A. E. *Johns Hopkins Hosp. Bull.* Baltimore, 1909, XIX, 274.
JANEWAY, T. C. *Arch. Int. Med.* Chicago, 1913, XII, 757.
KYLIN, E. *Acta med. Scandinav.* Stockholm, 1921, LV, 368.

Mahomed, F. A. *Guy's Hosp. Rep.* 1879, s. 3, xxiv, 363.
Marey. Travaux du Laboratoire. Paris, 1875.
Martin, C. J. *Brit. Med. Journ.* 1905, i, 865.
Poiseuille, J. L. M. "Recherches sur la force du cœur aortique," *Journ. de physiol.* Paris, 1828, viii, 272.
Riva-Rocci, S. *Gazz. med. di Torino,* 1897, xlviii, 161, 181.
van Leersum, E. C. "Old Physiological Experiments," *Janus,* Leyde, 1913, xviii, 325.
von Recklinghausen. *Arch. f. exper. Path. u. Pharm.* 1901, xlvi, 110.

Sphygmographs:

Burdon-Sanderson. Handbook of the Sphygmograph. London, 1867.
Dudgeon, R. E. The Sphygmograph. London, 1882.
Mackenzie, J. Study of the Pulse. 1902.
Mahomed, F. A. *Med. Times and Gaz.* 1872.
Vierordt, K. Die Lehre vom Arterienpuls. 1855.

The Electrocardiograph:

Burdon-Sanderson and Page. *Journ. Physiol.* Cambridge, 1879–80, ii, 384.
Lewis, T. "Obituary of Einthoven," *Proc. Roy. Soc.* B, 1928, vol. 102, p. v.
Oppenheimer and Rothschild. *Journ. Am. Med. Assoc.* 1917, lxix, 429; *Trans. Assoc. Am. Phys.* 1924, xxxix, 247.
Waller, A. D. *Phil. Trans.* 1889, clxxx, 169.

Auricular Flutter:

Drury, A. N. and Iliescu, C. C. *Heart,* London, 1921, viii, 171.
Hertz, A. F. and Goodhart, G. W. *Quart. Journ. Med.* Oxford, 1908–9, ii, 213.
Jolly, W. A. and Ritchie, W. T. *Ibid.* 1910–11, ii, 177.
Lewis, T. *Brit. Med. Journ.* 1921, i, 551.
Lewis, Feil and Stroud. *Heart,* London, 1920, vii, 191.
MacWilliam, J. A. *Journ. Physiol.* Cambridge, 1887, viii, 296.
Mines, G. R. *Ibid.* 1913, xlvi, 349.
Ritchie, W. T. *Proc. Roy. Soc. Edin.* 1905, xxv, 1085.

118   INSTRUMENTS OF PRECISION

Auricular Fibrillation:

ACKERMANN. *Deutsches Arch. f. klin. Med.* 1873, XI, 125.
ANDERSON, H. B. *Ann. Med. Hist.* N.Y. 1928, X, 47.
CUSHNY, A. R. and EDMUNDS, C. W. Studies in Pathology. Aberdeen, 1906. P. 95.
—— —— *Am. Journ. Med. Soc.* 1907, CXXXIII, 66.
DIXON, W. E. *Med. Mag.* London, 1907, XVI, 454.
EGGLESTON. *Am. Journ. Med. Sc.* Phila. 1920, CLX, 625.
FRASER, F. R. *Lancet*, London, 1922, ii, 703.
LEWIS, T. *Heart*, London, 1910, I, 306.
—— *Brit. Med. Journ.* 1921, i, 590.
LEWIS, T., DRURY, A. N., ILIESCU, C. C. and WEDD, A. M. *Heart*, London, 1922, IX, 207.
—— —— —— —— *Brit. Med. Journ.* 1921, ii, 514.
MACKENZIE, J. The Study of the Pulse. 1902. P. 209.
—— *Quart. Journ. Med.* Oxford, 1907–8, I, 39.
ROTHBERGER und WINTERBERG. *Pflüger's Arch. f. d. ges. Phys.* 1910, CXXXII, 243.
ROTHSCHILD, SACKS and LIBMAN. *Am. Heart Journ.* 1927, II, 356.
TRAUBE, L. *Charité-Ann.* 1851, 11.

Ventricular Fibrillation:

KRONECKER. Sitzungsb. d. Berl. Acad. 1884.
LUDWIG und HOFFA. *Ztschr. f. rat. Med.* 1850, IX, 107.
MACWILLIAM. *Brit. Med. Journ.* 1889, i, 6.

Paroxysmal Tachycardia:

BOUVERET. *Rev. de méd.* Paris, 1889, ix, 753.
COTTON, P. *Brit. Med. Journ.* 1867, i, 629.
GERHARDT, C. *Samml. klin. Vortr.* Leipzig, 1881 (inn. Med. No. 70), p. 1861.
HERRINGHAM, W. P. *Edin. Med. Journ.* 1897, N.S. I, 366.
LEWIS, T. *Heart*, London, 1909–10, I, 306.

History of Digitalis:

BALFOUR, G. W. Clinical Lectures on Diseases of the Heart and Aorta. Ed. 2. 1882. P. 339.
BLAKE, J. *Edin. Med. and Surg. Journ.* 1839, LI, 330.
BRUNTON, T. L. On Digitalis with some Observations on the Urine (Thesis 1866). London, 1868.

BRUNTON and MEYER. *Journ. Anat. and Physiol.* 1873, VII, 135.

CULLEN, W. A Treatise of the Materia Medica. 1789. Vol. II, p. 555.

CUSHNY, A.R. The Action and Uses in Medicine of Digitalis and its Allies. 1925. P. 208.

DARWIN, E. *Med. Trans. Roy. Coll. Phys.* 1785, III, 255.

DONALDSON and STEVENS. *Journ. Physiol.* Cambridge, 1883, IV, 165.

FERRIAR, J. Medical Properties of *Digitalis purpurea* or Foxglove. Manchester, 1799.

MACKENZIE, J. *Heart*, London, 1910–11, II, 284.

McKENZIE, D. The Infancy of Medicine. 1927. P. 173.

SAHLI. *Verhandl. Kongr. f. inn. Med.* 1901, XIX, 45.

VAQUEZ, H. *Arch. du mal du cœur, des vaisseaux, et du sang*, Paris, 1924, XVII, 545.

WYNN, H. W. *Birmingham Med. Rev.* 1926, N.S. I, 45.

IV

Physiological and Pathological Experiment

CLINICAL observation on the one hand and physiological and pathological research or experimental medicine on the other hand, though resembling each other to some extent, are not identical; pure observation of the natural history of disease, such as Hippocrates practised, does not include any interference with its course. Treatment, which is an attempt to alter the natural sequence of events, may be empirical, that is a more or less blind act derived from experience, or may be based on the reasoned results of experiment on animals. The repeated observation that a remedy, perhaps originally tried accidentally and become traditional, exerts a beneficial therapeutic effect is valuable, but often it lacks a sure foundation, being influenced by the shifting sands of the complex factors inherent in human biology.

Essential in all branches of medicine, in none except in neurology has experimental physiology been more inseparably connected with progress than in the cardiovascular system. Clinical observation alone, though in the hands of the greatest intellects, has laboured long and often ineffectually, but when aided and corrected by experimental control has rapidly brought about an advance in cardiological knowledge. This difference in the results given by these two ways—clinical observation and experiment—of obtaining new knowledge in medical science, which is so disappointing to the pure clinician that he may not unnaturally contest the statement, depends on the inherent potentialities of the two methods; in clinical observation the conditions cannot be arranged to meet the exact requirements as can be done in a laboratory. The clinical ward has been called the physician's laboratory, but obviously this phrase does not confer the same opportunities for exact determination of questions by the sharp-cut experiments available in the physiological laboratory. On the other hand, some care must be taken in transferring the results on animals to the more complex conditions in man. As disease, according to Claude Bernard's definition, is a physiological reaction in altered circumstances, it is obvious that the laws of these reactions can be much more surely established and the modifying circumstances varied and controlled by well-considered animal experiments. Further, animal experiments prepare the way for the application of somewhat similar methods to man, thus Stephen Hales' experiments on blood pressure find their clinical representatives in the modern sphygmomanometers, Marey's tambours, and Mackenzie's polygraph; the observations of electrical changes in muscular contraction, especially on the frog, "the Job of physiology", as being the animal most extensively used by physiologists (Bernard), eventually led up to the electrocardiograph. Thus, to quote the Presidential Harveian Oration of 1926, "the discoveries of the pure clinicians, remarkable as they were for the acuteness of their observation, were largely dependent on making use of the methods and apparatus of the laboratory in the investigation of clinical problems".

In 1845 the brothers E. F. and Ernst Heinrich Weber, repeating with the advantage of more exact physiological knowledge the experiments of R. Lower in 1669, showed that stimulation of the vagi slowed and inhibited the heart's action, and the accelerating effect of the sympathetic was pointed out in 1863 by von Bezold; it was then naturally assumed that the cardiac contractions depended on the activity of intracardiac ganglia and nerves, and were nervous in origin rather than merely controlled by the nervous system. This neurogenic hypothesis, though modified by Engelmann, eventually was superseded by the myogenic conception of the cardiac contractions as the result of the work of W. H. Gaskell (1847–1915), following J. G. Romanes' (1848–94) demonstration of the block that can be produced to the passage of contraction waves in medusae. Gaskell (1883) proved that the cardiac contractions arise in the muscular tissue independently of the nerves and ganglia, and that the auricles and ventricles have their own automatic rhythm, though normally obedient to the influence of the sinus. This was to some degree foreshadowed by Harvey's observation that if the ventricle of an eel or that of various fish is cut into pieces contractions continue to occur in the several portions. It must not be forgotten that the recognition in 1672 of muscular irritability by Harvey's fellow Caian, Francis Glisson (1597–1677), which was revived by Albrecht von Haller (1708–1777), who in 1757 stated that the cardiac contractions originated in the muscle, was the first step in the recent elucidation by Gaskell in physiology and in pathology by Lewis and others of cardiac problems.

Although in his second letter to Riolan in 1649 Harvey showed that he was familiar with local disturbances in the character of the cutaneous circulation, it was not until long after the great conception of the circulation as a whole was established that its local characters received special consideration. The effects of embolism, studied by Virchow (1846–56), and independently in this country by W. Senhouse Kirkes (1852), led, from the resulting lesions, to the realization of end-arteries in the kidney and brain on the one hand, and on the other hand to the recognition of the peculiarities of the circulation in the spleen, lung, and liver, the two last having nutrient arteries (bronchial and hepatic) in addition to the vessels (pulmonary artery and portal vein) conveying blood to be modified in those viscera.

Nearly fifty years ago Roy pointed out that the *splenic circulation* differs from that of other organs in the important particular that the force which drives the blood through the organ is not the arterial blood pressure, but chiefly, if not exclusively, the rhythmic contraction of the muscular fibres in the splenic capsule and trabeculae. Barcroft's observations suggest that in the spleen there are alternative circulations and that the blood of the large splenic artery may either (i) when not required elsewhere, as it is in the emergencies of exercise or haemorrhage, accumulate in the splenic pulp, there to undergo changes, or (ii) rapidly traverse a by-pass, and incidentally, like the bronchial arteries to the lungs and the hepatic artery to the liver, maintain the nutrition of the viscus. The blood stored in the spleen may contain as much as a quarter of the red cells and, as shown by Barcroft's experiments with CO poisoning, be practically cut off from the general circulation and so remain free from a poisoned state ruling elsewhere. Anoxaemia stimulates the smooth muscle fibres in the spleen and so drives out the resting blood; it thus, as Henry Gray (1854) pointed out, regulates the quantity and quality of the circulating blood. While serving as a reservoir the spleen also acts as a metabolic refinery for the red blood cells and a manufactory for the white cells. The resting blood in the spleen deposits any foreign matter, such as bacteria, protozoa, and cells of malignant growths, which may either be destroyed, the process being an immunological asset, or remain and by multiplying there account for the splenomegalies of chronic diseases, such as malaria, kala-azar, "splenic anaemia". As an important storehouse of reticulo-endothelial cells the spleen is concerned with the destruction of the red blood corpuscles, increasing their fragility by what Botazzi (1895) called its haemokatatonistic function, and plays an important part in the first stage of the transformation of effete haemoglobin into bilirubin.

Wearn's even more recent evidence that the blood in the coronary arteries has alternative circulations, either through the capillaries into the coronary sinus, as usually considered, or directly into the Thebesian or other veins and so into the cardiac cavities, is of obvious importance in connection with angina pectoris (*vide* p. 91).

These data have a bearing on the question of the reserve power of the organs, which in the past has been regarded as mainly or entirely quantitative in

character. Now it would appear that the reserve
power may also depend on the utilization of potential alternative courses of the circulating blood,
and that in pathological conditions compensatory
processes may maintain the reserve of an organ,
as has been mentioned in the case of the heart in
coronary obstruction, and is perhaps also shown
in the increased size of the hepatic artery in cirrhosis
of the liver. The variations in the state of the
capillaries—full or empty—in different areas of
the body, which Thomas Young clearly anticipated in his forgotten Croonian Lecture before the
Royal Society in 1810, have been recently brought
out by the work of Krogh, Lewis, Dale, and others.

A more accurate knowledge of the unit blood
supply of the kidney and liver is important so as
to understand the mechanism and distribution of
changes likely to result from blood-borne toxaemias
or septicaemias and from chronic vascular disease.
With the help of X-rays and a radio-opaque injection
mass, normal and pathological kidneys have been
investigated with results encouraging as regards
further knowledge about differences between arteriosclerotic and glomerular nephritis (Graham).

The coronary arteries are provided with vaso-con-
strictor nerves from the vagus, and vaso-dilator from
the sympathetic (Anrep). Adrenaline undoubtedly
dilates the coronary arteries of animals usually em-

ployed in laboratory experiments; accordingly
Büdingen, at the suggestion of Morawitz and Zahn,
treated cases of angina pectoris with hypodermic
injections of adrenaline, but the results were nega-
tive. Barbour (1912) found that the action of
adrenaline causes vaso-constriction of rings of
human coronary artery, thus differing from its
effects in laboratory animals, and with Prince showed
that in the monkey this difference also holds good,
the coronary arteries of these two species being
presumably supplied with constrictor fibres from
the true sympathetic. Reference has already (p. 125)
been made to the anatomical peculiarities of the
coronary circulation, namely, the alternative passage
of blood direct from the arteries to the Thebesian
or other veins, the capillaries being short circuited,
and to the possibility, when the orifices of both coronary arteries are slowly occluded, of a circulation in
the reverse direction, viz. from the Thebesian
vessels into the coronary arteries (Wearn).

Pulmonary circulation. The questions whether or
not the branches of the pulmonary artery (i) are
under the control of the vasomotor nerves, and
(ii) are acted upon by drugs in the same manner as
the systemic vessels, are obviously of practical
importance in connection with the causation and
treatment of haemoptysis and pulmonary oedema.
The need of an authoritative lead from physiology

on these points was very clearly expressed by James Andrew in his Harveian Oration of 1901. Vaso-motor innervation of the pulmonary vessels was denied until 1871 when Brown-Séquard, who on experimental grounds argued that lesions of the pons caused haemorrhages, and injuries of the medulla oblongata oedema of the bases of the lungs as a result of impulses transmitted through branches of the sympathetic leaving the cord in the upper dorsal region. Rose Bradford and Dean (1889, 1894) found that in the dog vasomotor nerve fibres derived from the upper dorsal nerves supply the pulmonary blood vessels, though the pulmonary vasomotor mechan-ism is poorly developed as compared with that regulating the systemic arteries. They also con-cluded that the pulmonary circulation is com-paratively independent of the systemic, and that alterations in the blood pressure of the latter must be so considerable as to interfere with the action of the cardiac valves and produce regurgitation before affecting the pulmonary blood pressure. On the other hand, Brodie and Dixon in 1904 denied the vasomotor control of the pulmonary circulation and in 1928 Dixon and Hoyle confirmed this. In the meanwhile Führer and Starling, using the heart-lung preparation, found a considerable degree of pulmonary vaso-constriction and a rise of pulmonary arterial pressure with adrenaline, and in 1905

François-Franck came to a similar decision. In a critical review of the extensive work on the subject Wiggers in 1921 concluded that reflex vasomotor effects on the pulmonary circulation must be regarded as probable rather than proved.

The intracranial circulation is remarkable for the rigid cranial cavity and the water-bed of the cerebrospinal fluid. Whether or not the nerves accompanying the cerebral vessels exert a vasomotor function has been repeatedly investigated, but with discordant results; Roy and Sherrington (1890), L. Hill (1896), and more recently Florey (1925) who found that the cerebral arteries and the cerebral ends of the capillaries react to mechanical, thermal, electrical, and chemical stimuli by contraction and dilatation, agree that there is not any evidence of nervous control over the cerebral vessels. On the other hand, the existence of active functional control of the cerebral vessels by vasomotor nerves has been supported by Claude Bernard (1858), Nothnagel (1867), Wiggers (1915), Forbes and Wolff (1928), and others. The experimental observations are of much interest in connection with the belief held by many clinicians that transient paralyses, such as occur without evidence of a gross lesion, may be due to spasm of the cerebral arteries analogous to that in Raynaud's disease. Osler (1911), in describing transient attacks of aphasia and paralysis in states of high blood pressure and arteriosclerosis, accepted the view put forward by Peabody (1891), W. Russell (1909), and others that they were due to transient spasm. Florey has thrown out the suggestion that possibly in pathological conditions, such as arteriosclerosis, an abnormal metabolic product which has not any effect on normal blood vessels, may produce spasm of damaged arteries.

The influence of the conditions of the cerebral circulation on the general blood pressure has been much discussed. Starling and Anrep (1925) showed that when imperfectly supplied with blood the vasomotor centre brings about a compensatory rise of blood pressure, thus confirming Cushing's earlier demonstration in 1901 that the vasomotor centre exerts a regulating influence whereby anaemia of the medulla oblongata is prevented when the intracranial pressure is increased above that in the cerebral vessels. This was supported by Bordley and Baker's (1926) observation that in arteriosclerosis a high blood pressure was definitely associated with sclerosis of the arterioles of the medulla; this, however, was contested by Keith, Wagener, and Kernohan, and Cutler's observations showed that gross vascular changes in the blood supply to the medulla were not responsible for blood pressure changes. Experimentally Florey, Marvin, and Drury (1928) found that lowering the blood pressure in the circle of Willis has not any influence upon the general blood pressure.

Ringer's pioneer work. The work carried on by Sydney Ringer (1835–1910) while actively engaged in hospital and consulting practice is remarkable in many respects for the circumstances in which it was done between 1870 and 1895, its simplicity, and the important influence it has exerted on scientific medicine. Ringer's fluid (1880–83) containing ions of chlorine, sodium, calcium and potassium in the form of inorganic salts in definite proportions has, except for magnesium salts which were added in 1910 by Tyrode, almost the same composition as sea-water. Ringer's fluid provides a substitute for the blood in so far as the activation of the living tissue is concerned, has been described as the foundation of a new branch of physiology, and with Locke's addition of glucose (1900) has facilitated experimental investigations in cardiology. His work is the basis of metabolic investigation in connection with calcium.

History of transfusion of blood. Although in accordance with the biblical text that "the blood is the life" the transference of blood from one individual to another was suggested, it only became rational and put into practice some time after Harvey's discovery of the circulation of the blood was published in 1628. In about 1650 Francis Potter, B.D., of Trinity

College, Oxford, and John Aubrey appear to have tried, but unsuccessfully, to transfuse one chicken from another, being impelled to this experiment by Ovid's story of Medea and Jason (Gunther). Richard Lower at Oxford, acting on the suggestion of Sir Christopher Wren, performed this experiment on dogs in 1665, as is recorded in John Ward's diary (D'Arcy Power), and published an account of it in the following year. The first authenticated transfusion of man with the blood of an animal (sheep) was performed in June 1667 by Jean Denys, Professor of Mathematics and Philosophy at Montpellier but not a medical man; after about fifteen other cases had been performed without any fatality (Cruchet, Ragot, and Caussimon) much opposition arose in France, and the Medical Faculty of Paris issued an injunction that it must not be performed without the approval of a member of their body. In November 1667 Lower and Edmund King transfused with sheep's blood an indigent Cambridge bachelor of divinity. But after this blood transfusion went out of fashion for a long time; in 1785 Busick Harwood urged, but did not perform, transfusion from animals to man, and in 1792 Russell transfused a boy for hydrophobia with lambs' blood (Keynes). In the nineteenth century Thomas Blundell (1790–1878) and other obstetricians performed transfusion on about 400 patients between

1818 and 1824; there was a revival of the procedure in Germany between 1860 and 1880, terminating with von Bergmann's monograph (1883), and contemporaneously Oré of Bordeaux between 1860 and 1876 transfused men from animals in 165 cases with one fatality only (Cruchet, Ragot, and Caussimon). But after this transfusion again sank into oblivion until George Crile in 1909 invented a suitable technique for transfusion from one human being to another, and the four blood groups in man were described (Jansky (1907) and Moss (1910)). The Great War rendered blood transfusion a well-recognized and routine method of treatment. Cruchet has insisted on the safety and other advantages of heterogenous, namely from animal to man, transfusion.

Intravenous medication. In 1656 Christopher Wren (1632–1723) injected wine and ale into the veins of a dog in the direction of the heart, and anticipated that this practice would be of use in medicine. This hope was not fully realized until after Ehrlich's salvarsan treatment was given to the world in 1910.

134 PHYSIOLOGICAL EXPERIMENT

REFERENCES

IV

BARCROFT, J. *Lancet*, London, 1926, i, 544.
BERNARD, C. An Introduction to the Study of Experimental Medicine. Transl. by H. C. Greene. New York, 1927. P. 115.
BOTAZZI, P. *Arch. ital. di biol.* Torino, 1895, XXIV, 462.
BRADFORD, J. ROSE. *Brit. Med. Journ.* 1926, ii, 719.
GASKELL, W. H. *Journ. Physiol.* Cambridge, 1883, IV, 43.
GLISSON, F. Tractatus de Naturae Substantiae energetica. 1672.
GRAHAM, R. S. *Bull. Ayer Clin. Lab.* Penna. Hosp. 1928, No. 11, p. 58.
GRAY, H. The Spleen. London, 1854.
HALLER, A. Elementa Physiologiae. 1757.
HARVEY, W. Willis' transl. of the *De Motu.* 1847. P. 28.
KIRKES, W. S. *Med.-Chir. Trans.* 1852, XXXV, 281.
ROMANES, J. G. *Phil. Trans.* 1875, CLXVI, 269.
ROY, C. S. *Journ. Physiol.* Cambridge, 1880–82, III, 203.
VIRCHOW, R. *Beitr. z. exper. Path. u. Physiol.* 1846, 2 Heft, 1.
WEARN, J. T. *Journ. Exper. Med.* 1928, XLVII, 293.

Coronary Arteries:

ANREP, G. V. *Physiol. Rev.* 1926, VI, 596.
BARBOUR, H. G. *Journ. Exper. Med.* 1912, XV, 404.
BARBOUR and PRINCE. *Ibid.* 1915, XXI, 330.
MORAWITZ und ZAHN. *Deutsches Arch. f. klin. Med.* 1914, CXVI, 388.
WEARN, J. T. *Journ. Exper. Med.* 1928, XLVII, 293.

Pulmonary Circulation:

BRADFORD, J. R. and DEAN, H. P. *Proc. Roy. Soc.* 1889, XLV, 369.
—— —— *Journ. Physiol.* 1894, XVI, 34.
BRODIE, T. G. and DIXON, W. E. *Journ. Physiol.* 1904, XXX, 476.
BROWN-SÉQUARD, C. E. *Lancet*, London, 1871, i, 6.
DIXON, W. E. and HOYLE, J. C. *Journ. Physiol.* 1928, LXV, 299.
FRANÇOIS-FRANCK. *Arch. de physiol.* 1905, XXVII, 744.
FÜHNER, H. and STARLING, E. H. *Journ. Physiol.* 1913, XLVII, 286.

Intracranial Circulation:

BORDLEY, J. and BAKER, B. M. *Bull. Johns Hopkins Hosp.* Baltimore, 1926, XXXVI, 320.
CUSHING, H. *Ibid.* Baltimore, 1901, XII, 290.
FLOREY, H. *Brain*, London, 1925, XLVIII, 43.
FLOREY, MARVIN and DRURY. *Journ. Physiol.* Cambridge, 1928, LXV, 204.
FORBES and WOLFF. *Arch. Neurol. and Psychiat.* Chicago, 1928, IX, 1057. (Full bibliography.)
HILL, L. The Physiology and Pathology of the Cerebral Circulation. London, 1896.
NOTHNAGEL, H. *Virchows Arch.* 1867, XL, 203.
OSLER, W. *Canad. Med. Assoc. Journ.* Toronto, 1911, I, 919.
PEABODY, G. *Trans. Assoc. Am. Phys.* Phila. 1891, VI, 170.
ROY and SHERRINGTON. *Journ. Physiol.* Cambridge, 1890, XI, 85.
STARLING, E. H. and ANREP, G. V. *Proc. Roy. Soc.* 1925, XCVII, B, 643.

Transfusion of Blood:

CRUCHET, R. *Brit. Med. Journ.* 1926, ii, 975.
CRUCHET, R., RAGOT, A. et CAUSSIMON, J. La transfusion du sang de l'animal à l'homme. 1928. P. 10.
GUNTHER, R. T. Early Science in Oxford, 1925, III, 127.
KEYNES, G. Blood Transfusion, Oxford Medical Publications. 1922, p. 9.
LOWER, R. *Phil. Trans.* 1666, I, 352.
POWER, D'A. *Trans. Med. Soc. Lond.* 1920, XLIII, 277.

INDEX OF AUTHORS

SUBJECT INDEX